In the Shadows: Living and Coping with a Loved One's Chronic Illness

David M. Luterman, D.Ed.
Professor, Communication Disorders
Emerson College
Boston, MA 02116

Jade Press
Box 822
Bedford, MA 01730

This book was manufactured in the United States of
America. Typography by The Type Shoppe, Inc. Printing
and binding by McNaughton & Gunn, Inc. Cover design by
Joseph Dieter, Jr. Book design by Sheila Stoneham.

Library of Congress Number 95-94103

Table of Contents

About the Author

David Luterman has been a Professor of Communication Disorders at Emerson College in Boston for the past 30 years. He has operated a parent-centered nursery for the families of newly diagnosed deaf children and has given numerous workshops throughout the United States and Canada. He is the author of five books: *Counseling Parents of Hearing Impaired Children* (1979, Little, Brown), *Counseling the Communicatively Disordered and Their Families* (1984, Little, Brown), Editor, *Deafness in Perspective* (1986, College-Hill Press), *Deafness in the Family* (1987, College-Hill Press), and *When Your Child is Deaf* (1991, York Press). He is a Fellow of the American Speech-Language-Hearing Association.

Acknowledgements

This book has been written over a ten year period, going through many metamorphoses in the process. In one sense this book can never be really finished as I am detailing in part, the process of living with someone I love who has a chronic, progressive illness. It is the story of me and my wife Cari, grappling with her disease, multiple sclerosis, and as such I am hopeful that there are more chapters to come.

An astonishingly large number and variety of people have helped me with this book. Many friends, colleagues, and relatives read and commented on portions of this book. Among the multitudes were: Elaine Adler, Dick Duprey, Mike Kittross, Peg Lahey, Helen Ross, Al and Kay Davis, Sue Colten, and my brother Barry and sister Arlene. Eileen Sussman, Louise Akillian and Cindy Z. were very helpful in finding people to interview. My children Alison, Daniel, Emily, and James were immensely helpful in reading portions of the book, contributing their experiences and supporting me. Nancy Platerborze was a very tough copy editor and supporter. Judy Macadoo and Liz Bezara, librarians bar none, were able to find any and all references I requested (and some were obscure). The faculty research committee of Emerson supported me generously in my efforts to get the manuscript typed and published. Since I write my books on my kitchen table with ball point pen on yellow legal paper I have need for a good typist. Over the years I have been blessed with a slew of them—Melanie Ranson, Susan Lipsky, Dan Petche, Ann Solomon, and last, but among the best, Christine Starratt. They were all unfazed by my frequent requests, able to read my scrawl, and were competent in all that they did. To Elinor Hartwig, who saw the book through the publication process, I am forever grateful. And, of course, Cari who did so much to make this book possible: without her help and indeed without her illness, this book would not have been possible.

This book is dedicated to the friends
who came so faithfully every day
to work with Cari
on her exercise program
and to Steve and Sol
who did not live to see this publication.

Life is not a matter of holding good cards,
but of playing a poor hand well.
—Robert Louis Stevenson

Author's Note

All the interview data reported in this book were recorded by me during spontaneous sessions with the healthy family members whom, in the text, I call the shadow spouse or sometimes the co-disabled. I only had to ask a few leading questions and their stories would come tumbling out. As much as possible in the text, I wanted them to tell their own stories; these are generally isolated and lonely people who do not get much attention. They are grateful for the chance to talk to someone; they need to be listened to. I also changed or eliminated any names that might identify the participants. These people were selected solely on their willingness to participate in this project, and as such, they are not necessarily representative of all able-bodied family members, although I think their stories are fairly typical. They are courageous people to whom I am grateful for allowing me to share their lives, if only for a short while.

Introduction

According to family therapists, a family is a system, by which it is meant that all of the parts of a family are interconnected in such a way that cause and effect cannot be distinguished. When one part of a family system is "damaged" in some way, then every part is affected: this means that when one member of a family has a chronic, progressive illness, all members of the family have it. This idea of the interconnectedness of family has had much meaning to me in both my professional life, where I have been working intimately for over 30 years with the families of newly diagnosed deaf children, and, more pointedly in my personal life where my wife, Cari, has been diagnosed as having multiple sclerosis (MS).

Multiple sclerosis is an autoimmune disease in which the T cells of the immune system attack the myelin sheath that covers the nerves of the central nervous system, forming scar tissue or plaques that interfere with the transmission of nervous impulses. The disease typically manifests itself in young adults. The cause, as of now, is unknown and there is no known cure. The type my wife has is chronic, progressive multiple sclerosis in which the disease slowly feasts on the margins of her motor abilities, causing a slow but inexorable decline in her neurological functioning.

Twenty-seven years ago when my wife was in her early thirties she complained of a "fullness" in her right eye and some loss of peripheral vision. She had suffered a blow on the head a few days earlier and we attributed the eye problem to the head trauma. When the blurred vision persisted, she went for an eye examination. The ophthalmologist alarmed us by his concern but did not make a diagnosis; fortunately, he referred us directly for a neurological examination. The neurologist told us at that time that my wife either had an optic neuritis that would clear up by itself, or it was the first manifestation of multiple sclerosis. We, very consciously, chose to believe that it was optic neuritis and promptly "forgot" the MS possibility.

The blurred vision cleared up and we proceeded to live our very busy lives managing our family and two careers. We had our fourth child and life went on. In retrospect, there were several little things that we ignored in the intervening years such as Cari complaining that she couldn't walk easily down the mountain on our hikes, or hit a ping-pong ball well enough to play the game anymore. (I can remember vividly her complaining, "If they only had a name for it.") Leakage from her bladder was attributed to the four pregnancies. Finally, ten years after the initial tentative diagnosis, she began to develop head tremors and weakness in her leg while jogging, which we could ignore no longer. We returned to the neurologist, who, after several more tests, confirmed the diagnosis of chronic, progressive multiple sclerosis. When he told us, he added that this was the most optimistic diagnosis he could give at that time, and I remember thinking I wouldn't want his job. I still don't!

As of this writing, 17 years after the confirmation of the diagnosis, the disease has slowly and silently progressed and Cari has steadily declined in her abilities. She has changed from an able-bodied woman who could run 10K races easily to a woman in a wheelchair barely able to transfer from her chair to the bed, the car, or the toilet. And I have changed from a rather free-wheeling spouse with a great deal of personal space, able to pursue my professional career with much support from my wife, to a much more restricted family member who has been increasingly assuming more and more responsibility for maintaining the family homeostasis.

Because of the disease we have had to make considerable modification in our home and family life. We remodeled our home, adding a room on the first floor to serve as our bedroom with a handicapped accessible bathroom and a lift into the house which by-passes the stairs. We modified our station wagon to accommodate a three-wheeled electric scooter and put hand controls on the steering wheel so that Cari could continue to drive. Because of her difficulties in transferring to the driver's seat, we have recently purchased a van that will transport her but is not modified for her to drive. As of this writing it is unlikely that she will ever drive again and this is a big blow. Her bladder difficulties have increased and the fatigue she experiences, which is an almost universal symptom of MS, makes her sometimes not want to get out of bed in the morning (Cari denies that this is MS fatigue but says rather it is the inertia and difficulty she experiences in getting her muscles to move).

Despite her increasing disability, Cari has managed to complete the job of raising our children (our last child graduated from college three years ago), do her share of the housework, and work part-time as a tutor with both children and adults for whom English is a second language. In these past 17 years, she has managed to complete a Master's degree, continues to take courses, and serves on several committees within our town (one of which is the Enablement Committee which seeks to make the town more accessible to all, including people with disabilities). Recently she has won an award from a community college as someone who has made a difference. She generally has dealt with her disease with forthrightness and has not let it interfere with living life to the fullest. She is much more active than I and she has taught me much about courage; I both love and admire her greatly; and in many respects, despite the ravages of this disease, we both consider ourselves lucky.

This book, however, is not about her or her disease—at least not directly. It is about me, or about any spouse who is living with someone who has chronic, progressive illness. These are people who live in the penumbra cast by the spotlight of the disease, the people in the shadows, whom I sometimes refer to as the co-disabled. They are the ones who fetch and carry, who transport and worry, and are constantly assuming greater responsibilities in their marriages, yet they receive almost no professional or personal attention. These are the people who cool their heels in waiting rooms while the patient goes through endless tests. These are the ones who are juggling finances and baby sitters. The co-disabled are the ones who must learn to live with ambiguity, uncertainty, and ever changing levels of disability in their loved one. They live with the knowledge that for them, as for their spouse, the worst is probably yet to be.

My wife and I have been lucky; we have been treated very well. Her disease was diagnosed accurately, which is generally not the rule in multiple sclerosis, and our neurologist, to his everlasting credit, always included me in all examinations and discussions. Yet it is the rare individual who looks at me and asks me how I am doing; almost everyone wants to know, and it's understandable, how my wife is. Occasionally though, I need some attention. When I do ask for attention, it is always tinged with guilt as though I do not have the right to complain. People almost always look at the person in the wheelchair, seldom at the person pushing it.

For the past several years, I have been facilitating well-spouse support groups for the MS Society. At one meeting, a wife introduced herself by saying, "I, too, have had MS for 17 years; only nobody knows it," and everybody in the room nodded their head in understanding. Another wife put it so well when she said, "In this concert, I will always be second violin." And while no one would want the first chair, there are times when attention needs to be directed to the spouse and other family members. There are several books available that are by and for the person with the disease (my wife would never let me say "victim"), yet there is little literature on the well family members, with the exception of a recent notable book by Strong.[1] My own personal and professional solution to a problem is to study it—to find out as much as I can about it. This is my own means of trying to get some measure of control over the problem. The strategy has served me well over the years and so I set about reviewing the literature and interviewing well family members of the chronically ill in preparation for this book. This book then is a result of both my personal experience and professional investigations. In the course of researching this book I have met some remarkable and courageous people who were in very difficult situations.

Among them were:

A young woman, joining an MS spouse group because she did not know whether to continue her courtship with her lover who was recently diagnosed with MS.

A man who has been very painfully talking with his mother, newly-diagnosed with cancer and care-taker of her husband who has Alzheimer's disease, about the possibility of murder/suicide.

A healthy spouse of a man with MS reeling from the knowledge that her daughter has just been diag-nosed as having MS also.

The wife of a professional man who has been pre-vented by her husband from talking to anyone about his MS for fear of losing patients.

The guilt burdened husband who just put his very disabled wife of 35 years into a nursing home so that he could now "have a life."

All of these people and many others were not prepared for the awesome responsibility that chronic illness presents, yet they were able to deal with these problems in a way that promoted their own personal growth. I have come to see these chronic illnesses not only as tremendous stressors but also as powerful teachers—perhaps they are the teachers because they are also the stressors.

This is a book that will try to tell the story of the co-disabled who are living with family members who have a chronic, progressive illness. I hope to convey chronic, progressive illness through the eyes of the healthy family members, and to provide for the reader a perspective from the inside of the family. I hope to be able to offer help for those families in understanding the illness and in coping with its ramifications.

I have interviewed co-disabled family members of

five diffferent illnesses, all of which I think are illus-
trative of the general problems confronting the well
family members of a chronically ill person: multiple
sclerosis, diabetes, Alzheimer's disease, rheumatoid
arthritis, and lupus. Descriptions of each of these diseases may be found in the appendix. At first glance it
may seem that these are disparate diseases, but there
is a universality to the coping process of chronic, progressive illness—under the disability skin, we are all
brothers and sisters.

All of the diseases described in this book present
problems of diagnosis. I have seldom met a family in
which there wasn't some delay in the diagnosis of the
disease. For us it took ten years from the first symptoms to the definite diagnosis. This is not necessarily
a failure of the medical profession so much as it is a
reflection of the insidious and variable nature of these
diseases. Onset is invariably very slow and very easy
to blame on some minor problem; it is when all the
conventional treatments fail and symptoms worsen in
the face of standard medical interventions that patient and doctor begin the long journey of trying to
eliminate possibilities until they are left with only one
probability.

These also are diseases in which the etiology is
unknown and for which there is no known cure. They
are chronic and progressive and, as such, they violate
everything we know or think we know about disease.
Illness for most of us means either recovery or death.
We can prepare ourselves for either eventuality, pre-
ferably the former rather than the latter. There is
nothing in life, though, that helps us prepare for
chronic, progressive illness. We are told that despite
the best of medical treatment the patient probably
will get worse and will have this disease for the rest

of his or her life, which in many cases can be a great many years since almost all of these diseases have their onset in young adulthood.

Society offers us no rituals, such as those that surround death, to assuage the pain we feel, yet to live with chronic illness is to experience a succession of little deaths. It is a dying by inches, an ongoing funeral that society does not recognize. These diseases were selected because they are fairly common chronic illnesses currently plaguing our society; it is estimated that there are 30 million Americans who have dysfunctions due to chronic illness, and that 80 percent of our health care facilities are now devoted to chronic disease. It is also estimated that currently the cost of dementia alone is 40 billion dollars and this figure is rapidly increasing as our society ages, and as we find treatments that transform previously terminal diseases to chronic ones.[3]

In this book I want to tell the families' stories because it is a seldom told story of people struggling with the problem of constant adjustment; the co-disabled face a frightening future that is only dimly seen through the mist of medical uncertainty. It is also, I hope, a testament to the strength and the capacity of people to grow and find joy and meaning in difficult situations. I have found the people I have met in the course of researching for and writing this book to be marvelous monuments to the resilience of human nature. This book then is written by, about, and for the people who are in the shadows of chronic, progressive illness.

CHAPTER I

Those Unruly Feelings

As I sit in Temple with Cari perched next to me on her scooter, watching women actively going up and down to the altar, unbidden into my mind comes the thought "I want a wife who can walk." I am startled by the intensity of my wish and the ensuing pain that I feel. I am usually able to keep such thoughts and feelings at bay by working actively to solve "the problem" or by assiduously denying it. But on this occasion neither strategy worked as I was caught in a contemplative mood—the feelings of pain and loss just washed over me, and I know that I just have to allow the feelings to run their course. There is no way anyone who is living with someone with chronic, progressive illness can not feel the pain of the loss. I remember the wife of a blind, diabetic who was in tears as she started to tell me about her life and she kept saying " I am doing this badly"—I kept assuring she was doing it just right. The loss, and it is a very intense loss, is of the dream of the expected future. Cari and I at this point in our lives fully expected to be living a vigorous middle age life as the children were grown, debts were paid, and our dog had died. With our health, what a marvelous time of life for us! Every once in a while, at times when I least expect it, the loss of that future overwhelms me and I grieve. The pain of that loss will never go away.

Chronic diseases usually begin insidiously, that is, the first symptoms are mild and easily explained. For example, Cari's eye problem could be explained as an optic neuritis brought on by the head trauma and many of the first symptoms of arthritis and lupus are seen as the normal aches and pains of increasing age, as are the memory lapses of early Alzheimer's disease. With these diseases, however, the symptoms persist and intensify in the face of self-administered conventional treatment or remedies recommended by a physician. It is a rare family that receives a rapid and accurate diagnosis of the disease. More often than not, the chronically ill go through several physicians and diagnoses before the disease is diagnosed accurately. During this period of uncertainty, we are on an emotional roller coaster: elation when we receive an optimistic diagnosis and despair when the prescribed remedy does not work and/or new symptoms appear, as they inevitably do. It is almost a relief when we get a definite diagnosis. I remember the dread and fear I felt when we went back to the neurologist. I can describe that scene in detail, it is etched forever in my mind—but oddly enough there was also a sense of relief as now her vague symptoms had a name and the enemy had a face. Multiple sclerosis is almost always difficult to diagnose.

Here is Barbara's account of that significant life turning-point when the diagnosis was made after two years of searching for a cause of her husband's symptoms:

But it was so hard just getting somebody to know what your symptoms mean; we searched for two years. Just before we went to the doctor with the myelogram, Henry thought he was going crazy, that it was a real mental problem, because these things were happening but they were telling us these things couldn't be. So when we found the specialist and she told us it was MS, we were almost relieved because at least we knew, or thought we knew, what we were dealing with. At least now it had a name. But the night of the test when we came home, I remember we were in bed, I remember thinking to myself, that if I hug him hard enough, maybe it will go away. I wanted to protect him so badly from the whole thing, and of course you can't. Actually he took it pretty well, although I don't think either of us knew what was involved, what it meant, and how it was going to affect our lives. The mental relief was very good for him to finally know that he does have something concrete, that it is not all in his mind. Maybe some people don't want to know what they have to deal with, like cancer patients, but we both wanted to know.

Lupus is also difficult to diagnose and the diagnostic process in and of itself is a nightmare as we can see here. Here in much more detail is the diagnosis of Lupus as seen through John's eyes:

It started five years ago. My wife was getting ready for her family to come for Thanksgiving dinner. The day after Thanksgiving she woke up, and she had a stiff neck and thought she must have pulled something, or did too much. By the following Monday, it had gotten quite stiff, so she went to our local doctor, and he agreed that she probably pulled something. He told her to put some heat on it and a neck collar on. If things aren't better in two or three days, come and see him. Two, three days went by, and she got progressively worse. She couldn't raise her shoulder so he sent her to an orthopedic doctor who did x-rays and blood tests—couldn't find anything wrong. Thought it might be an internal muscle or something. If it didn't get better to come back and see him and he'd give her a shot of cortisone and see what that does. She got worse; she couldn't turn her head or lift her arm, and went back to see him.

In the meantime, he had gotten back blood tests which had indicated a high sediment rate. He said, "I'm not going to give you cortisone. This is a different problem; it could be rheumatoid arthritis." He sent us to a doctor in Connecticut who ran a whole series of tests, sent us back home and put her on cortisone. This was now early December. From that

point on she started going downhill rapidly; it moved to all
the other joints. We lived in a split level ranch so there
were about eight steps to go up, two different levels, so she
couldn't even make those. I would have to carry her up and
down the stairs half the time, then I would also have to
wake her early in the morning and stick her in the bathtub
so that she could soak for half an hour before she had to get
the kids up. She could then get them up, get their lunches
and off to school, and then she'd go back to bed. During all
this time, back to the doctor, probably every third day—
hurting enough so she couldn't do it herself—plus I was concerned enough so that I wanted to go with her. Christmas
was horrible, although we got through it. About the middle
of January they put her in the hospital, ran a whole series of
tests on her, did a couple of biopsies, came back, and they
still couldn't tell what it was. So we were still seeing our
doctor once a week. He was playing around with cortisone—
sometimes it helped, sometimes it didn't. All this time she's
in a lot of pain; she cannot do all the normal things of cooking, washing dishes, etc. She's not very happy with herself—
she's scared to death. I'm certainly pretty upset—certainly
getting a rude awakening that I had always thought the
medical profession had gotten very scientific and could tell
us exactly what was going on—rapidly now reaching the
point where I realized that they *don't* know, damn well, what
was going on! Come to the second week of February and we
went away for the winter vacation with the kids. We were
there about two days, and she had started out with a sore
throat; it just got progressively worse. So finally I bundled
her into the car and took her to the local hospital. They heard
her litany of what had gone on in the past two months. They
became uncooperative; took a quick strep test and hustled
us out of there. I don't think they wanted to touch this with
a ten foot pole.

It went on, still having real trouble getting up and down
the stairs and getting anything done; she was mainly in bed.
She was very depressed and still hurting very badly. Our
doctor's reaction was that sometimes the hurt can be the
result of depression and psycho-induced, and did we want to
put her on valium? She didn't really want to go on it, but
then we thought, maybe you need to relax a bit and you

should try it. So we put her on a small dose of valium which helped a little bit; it made her easier to get along with and not quite so prone to emotional outbursts.

Then she developed severe pain in her side, took her to the doctor, he diagnosed pleurisy, put her to bed for the next week and a half. She was in bed most of the time because of the pain and because of the pleurisy. In the meantime, I had to take a business trip so my mother-in-law and sister-in-law came up to take care of Joan while I was away. They got terribly upset by Joan's condition. When I got in, my mother-in-law was in a complete tizzy. Joan was in terrible shape. She did not look good, she couldn't swallow, she couldn't eat. She complained that she hadn't eaten in two days. She couldn't drink liquids. I got the flashlight and looked in her mouth. The back of her mouth and throat were completely inflamed; bright fiery red with great big white lesions on it. I thought about it for a minute and then said, "O.K. kid, you're going to the hospital." We were very lucky, we had an excellent resident who jumped right into the thing. We were in the emergency room until about 1:30 in the morning while they ran every kind of test that they could think of. He was in consultation with three or four other doctors. They were running tests for the next week to ten days. A week later I walked into the hospital, the doctor called me aside and said, "Now I have some very personal questions to ask. What are you and your wife's sexual preferences, and do you know anything about AIDS?" The reason they were leaning that way is that there was just an absolute breakdown of her immune system. Finally, two days later, they realized it wasn't AIDS. They had gotten back the anti-DNA (ANA test) test which was terribly elevated, which really was a strong marker for SLE. So now we knew it was lupus. So then the doctor told me, "Just remember that almost anything that you can read anywhere about lupus is not true. If it was written over five years ago, it is out-of-date." So I still went to the library and got every damn piece of paper I could get my hands on. And in the case of lupus, it is extremely bad. Most of the writings in the early seventies said that you had about of 5% chance for five years. At least the doctor told me that that wasn't something to focus on; that survival was much better than that.

So they finally had her diagnosed as SLE. This was five months after the first pain and any number of doctors and examinations. She had been on massive doses of cortisone, antibiotics, and whole numbers of other things which we were now tapering down. She was now getting strong enough so that she was wanting to get out of the hospital and I was trying to get her to stay until she was sure she was well, because I knew I couldn't cope with her and the kids at the same time. She was also told that she couldn't get out until she could walk, so every day, twice a day, we would go down the hall and walk up and down the stairs to the next floor. She was getting better and maybe they were going to let her out the next day. I went home-six o'clock in the morning, the telephone rang. The voice said, "This is Mrs. so and so from CCU (Critical Care Unit), and last night your wife was moved down here because she has a very low blood pressure so we could monitor her. We didn't want you to go to an empty room." I said "Thank you" and hung up. I think at that point I was terribly overwhelmed and just laid there and sobbed for about fifteen minutes, and then I got our neighbors to watch the kids and I went to the hospital. Luckily by 1:00 everything was fine and they put her back in her room, and a day and a half later, they let her out.

As with John and Barbara, that diagnostic process for me and Cari was a mind numbing nightmare. No matter how prepared I thought I was for the diagnosis it still came as a jolt and I cannot recall much of what was said after the diagnosis was made—and it certainly took a long time before the implications sunk in. But I am convinced that, at this time, we need the psychological protection of shock and of the denial that follows shortly thereafter, to get through that day and over the very difficult times ahead, which we can only dimly sense. Shock is a divorcement of self from a situation ("I can't believe this is happening to me"). You feel that there is no connection between your head and your emotions. One spouse described her reactions to being told by the doctor that her husband had Alzheimer's disease as feeling that she was both on stage and seated in the audience observing her own performance. Another spouse described it as "walking through someone else's nightmare."

The feeling of shock is one of complete calmness, as though everything was happening in slow motion and to someone else. When you are in shock, you are able to move and to act, but are not yet ready to fully accept the diagnosis. Unfortunately, the mistake many professionals make is that of trying to give information too soon to people in a state of shock, and when this happens, it only leads to more anxiety and more confusion. You nod your head and may interject some appropriate questions or comments but the information is literally going in one ear and out the other. This is a necessary part of protecting yourself emotionally from devastating information that you are not ready to process. Another feeling that resembles shock is, in actuality, a kind of emotional exhaustion that happens to people who have undergone a series of emotionally stressful events as one often does with chronic illness. When a succession of bad or stressful things happen, to defend itself, the mind becomes almost numb. Where you might have previously responded with anxiety and worry, now you respond with resignation. There comes a point when the psychological energy has been depleted and there is nothing left. This is evident in John's narrative as he and his wife went through their series of misdiagnoses. It is not uncommon to see co-disabled at the end of their psychological tether in the early stages of the diagnostic process. Very often, the well spouse's apparent lack of response is misunderstood by professionals and is interpreted as a lack of concern, rather than the psychological exhaustion it is. Shock is often misunderstood and confused with indifference.

For the shadow spouse, the world has turned upside down in the space of the few minutes it took the physician to give a name to all those nagging, vaguely defined symptoms that the ill spouse was exhibiting. Now you are truly within the shadows; and even though it is still the same person who walked into the doctor's office with you, you will never be able to look at him or her in the same way again. You have lost your spouse. You also lost the life you thought you were going to have.

Denial also comes in early in the grief process and I have found that it persists throughout. At the simplest level it is Cari turning to me and saying "I can't believe this is us. What am I doing in this wheelchair?" At more complex levels, denial becomes a refusal to give into the demands of the disease. As such, it is not a bad response as it enables us to survive in the face of terrible events. In fact, none of the feelings described in this chapter are bad. I have had to learn that feelings just are. I never have to be responsible for how I feel but rather for how I behave.

Early in my professional career I was an audiological consultant for the Veterans Administration on a project involving testing survivors of the Spanish American War. At that time these men were well into their eighties and were declared totally disabled by the VA so that they could be tested in all aspects of their physical and mental functioning at government expense. This was one of the first studies on aging ever completed. One of the findings that emerged early in the study was the extent to which these men practiced denial. For example, our protocol for the hearing evaluation was an interview during which we asked the men how they thought they heard. After the third or forth repeat of the question, shouting it louder each time, invariably the answer was "fine." We had to throw out the question because we rarely got an answer other than "fine" despite the obvious evidence that they could not hear. What we did find, however, was that when these men began to admit and give in to their infirmities they invariably stopped participating in the study and they often died shortly afterward. So denial has its merits and I think is a necessary component of the process of coming to grips with the significant loss we are all facing for both us and our spouses. It enables us to get through the day, and by slowly yielding, denial enables us to accept, in pieces, what we are ready to deal with.

The next emerging emotion is usually the feeling of being overwhelmed and inadequate: in short being just plain scared. As denial slowly yields, this is the feeling that invades your bedroom at three A.M. as you lie sleepless next to your spouse. You ask such questions as "How can I possibly cope with the enormous responsibility of seeing my spouse through the disease? Will I have the psychological and physical resources to cope?" The fear is overwhelming; it is the fear of the unknown. For many spouses, at this point, the answer seems to be "No" and they physically leave or psychologically disappear into the woodwork; for others, it is a tremulous "Yes" and they stay, but are constantly re-evaluating their choice. I know of no spouse who does not wonder why they are staying and feel doubt about their ability to stay the course. We live with constant fear as the disease progresses.

Cari's disease process has been very slow and it is usually difficult to see any change on a week-to-week or month-to-month basis. Every once in a while though she has a mini-exacerbation in which she gets notably worse and then slowly recovers. We cannot fathom what triggers these exacerbations but they seem to be a portent of things to come; as she gradually seems to ratchet down to the state she was in when she had the exacerbation. This past summer as she was going to bed she discovered she could not move. She woke me up and I had to toilet her, undress her, put on her nightgown, and lift her dead weight into bed—a process that took the better part of an hour and that totally exhausted me. A few hours later she awoke me with the horrific request to "Please turn me over" as she was in the same position in which I had left her earlier in the night. I often think that this is our future and it terrifies me.

I cut a feature article from the *Boston Globe* about a devoted husband of 43 years living with his wife who has Alzheimer's disease. His day is devoted entirely to caring for his wife. The picture accompanying the article shows him holding his wife's hand with a look compounded of exhaustion, fear, and tenderness. She has the vacant stare of the advanced Alzheimer patient and I wonder if something like that is not in my future. His face haunts my dreams as I wonder about the depredations and difficulties to come. The caption for that picture is "Love's Loneliest Test." And I think the writer caught and documented the most poignant feeling that the well spouse feels: loneliness. Nobody really knows what it is like to live with someone you love who has a chronic progressive illness. I can only partially share my feelings with my family—I feel that my pain burdens them and I don't want to complain. Dear friends listen for a while but it gets boring for me and perhaps for them and I don't ever want to seem to be wallowing in self pity, which is so easy to do. There are always the few boors I have encountered who imply by their responses that I have no right to my grief because, after all, Cari has the disease. The only people who seem to understand are fellow shadow spouses and I feel most free in company with them. No matter what, though, there is nothing that alleviates the loneliness that I feel for any length of time. The problem is that the person I would most like to share my pain with is the cause of it. There is nobody to share the pain and responsibility the way a spouse would. And while Cari and I have good communication about her illness, I find that when I do share some of how I'm feeling, this increases her feelings of guilt and also fear that I might leave. So I have learned generally to keep a lid on my feelings and pick my times to unburden myself carefully. Every once in a while the intense feelings creep up on me as they did in Temple.

Underlying all the tension co-disabled spouses feel is the fear that the disease is progressing. The husband of an arthritic woman responds with anxiety when his wife complains of a twinge, which might very well herald the arrival of some further progression of the disease or just a pain from sitting in one position too long. It is so hard to sort out what is a normal feature of aging and what might be a herald of progression, so that everybody responds with alarm to any false step and the fear begins to reverberate anew. The world is no longer a safe place; you have lost the sense of invulnerability and of comfort. The environment is full of alarms and fears for me.

There is a great deal of fear, especially when I look ahead. When I feel like indulging in self pity, I can easily conjure up an image of me in a doddering old age barely able to push a wheelchair and wonder-

ing who or what agency will take care of us. There is
the constant fear I have that I might get sick; then
how would our family function? There is also the fear
that I might die first; then who would take care of
Cari? It often feels like we are in some kind of hell
without knowing what the original sin was.

I guess my biggest fear, and one seldom articulated, is that one of our children would get MS. I
don't know how I could handle that emotionally. Almost all disability couples who have children worry
about the health of their children. I know my wife
would respond with guilt that she somehow caused
this to happen. She seems to take responsibility for
all the bad genes the kids have and for everything
else bad, for that matter. There isn't much guilt to go
around when she is in the vicinity. I know my feelings
would be profound anger and despair. In the meantime, it is a quiet fear that I harbor which emerges
sometimes when I least expect it to. It is always there
whenever any of our children tell me they are not
feeling well. Sometimes it is articulated by our children and I try to reassure them but, in actuality, it is
myself I am trying to reassure, and I know I really
can't. That risk is there and there are no reassur-
ances; chronic, progressive illness can happen to anybody, and family members are a bit more susceptible
than the general population.

For many, the fear is also economic. How can the
family survive if the well spouse becomes the sole
support? This is almost always a serious problem
when the husband is ill, because wives are less likely
to earn a salary comparable to their husbands. There
is almost always economic hardship with chronic illness: there are appliances to buy, doctor's fees to pay,
and supportive services to purchase. Social agencies

are not always responsive to the needs of families with disability. It is uncertain at this writing whether the health care legislation will include provisions for long-term care—a daunting financial prospect we all face in an uncertain future. If the disease progresses as it has, Cari will require care that will be beyond my capacity to provide—nursing home costs are astronomical now and increasing almost daily. Will we have to use all of our accumulated wealth to provide care for her? I have already had to mortgage my secure, early retirement to renovate the house. At this point, we would have had a paid-up mortgage. Almost every disability family I have met is burdened by economic worries.

The fear and grief we feel serves to intensify all other feeling. Unfortunately the feeling that emerges very early and that serves to mask the others is anger. The anger becomes a useful channel for pent-up frustration and it very easily masks the fear. An angry spouse is often a scared spouse. This is the anger that occurs whenever a new symptom appears— the anger I feel when a new ineptitude is revealed as when another cup is broken and I want to shout, "Don't touch this! I can do it. Why do you have to be so clumsy?" Or the fury I feel when I trip over her wheelchair in our now too crowded kitchen. In reality I am asking, "Why do you have to have this disease?" There are the mornings I don't want to wake up because of the dread I feel that a new problem will confront me. There are many days and times when I silently scream "Don't tell me of another symptom!" This is the guilt, causing rage that silently accumulates, like equity in a house, and bursts forth when least expected and is seldom acknowledged for what it is. What I have to keep in mind is that I am mad at the situation and the disease, not Cari, but it does not always play out that way, and my outbursts tend to frighten and diminish her.

Here is how one couple worked it out.

> We got to a point where I could say to him, "I hate you. I hate you for being sick." There is so little we could do. We did so little anyway; we didn't socialize much really, and now we don't socialize at all. And he looks at me and says, "I know, I hate me for being sick, too." And then I'd get over it.

There is also the terrible anger, almost akin to rage, that comes from feelings of helplessness and impotence. It is the feeling that you can't do anything to take the pain and hurt of this disease away from someone you love. This is the sort of rage that leads to putting a fist through a door or kicking a cat, and anybody who crosses your path and looks at you the least bit cross-eyed had best watch out. There is the rage and anger you feel because you have no control. If you do happen to have a good day, it's not because you planned it that way. One young husband remarked, "I really resent this. I work hard all day, come home to an exhausted wife and two kids, and have to clean up and make supper and get the kids to bed and console my wife. I am exhausted and angry. Who can I get mad at? My wife doesn't want this any more than I do." Oh, how nice it would be if we could find a villain and slay him, but he doesn't exist. There is no one or nothing to get mad at, so you seethe with anger. Anger also gives way to bewilderment as I, like Cari, wonder how this happened to us.

Another source of anger is the loss of control we feel. It is the restrictions that are now put on our lives by the disease. Going out, for example, becomes a major chore as we have to scout out whether the restaurant or theater is handicapped accessible and where the toilets may be—this is so easy for other people and used to be so for us. Planning vacations are equally difficult as we have just a narrow range of choices and even though we can and do go out, a lot more work and effort is required and we are faced continually with a limited range of options. It is not even that we might want to go, it is that we have no choice about it!

All of the chronic, progressive illnesses generate a great deal of uncertainty about the future. Physicians tell us, in effect, that there is no cure and that they cannot predict its course. Many physicians try to present a more optimistic scenario than they might feel and usually the literature provided by agencies devoted to the particular disease also try to present an optimistic frame. At heart we know that no one can predict the future as no one could have foretold that we would have the disease in the first place. So I tend to mistrust the prognostications and view the future when I choose to look at it, with a great deal of uncertainty. And when I take a long-range view—fear.

This means that we all must learn to live with uncertainty, fear of the future, and always a feeling of being powerless, in the face of advancing symptoms.

The husband of a woman who has lupus:

You keep fighting. You keep hoping she gets into remission, but the pain keeps coming. She'll be sitting there and all of a sudden you see her screwing up her face, because all of a sudden somewhere deep inside her hip the pain has started and that may last five minutes and go away or it may last twenty-four or thirty-six hours and go to her knee or anywhere else. It is the unknowing—where are we going from here. The lucky thing is it's been five years now and we've been relatively free of these problems, other than the aches and pain and tremendous fatigue. But in all cases, it is always in the back of your mind, "Is this going to be the time when it is going to hit her and flare up?"

Guilt is another feeling that is almost always present in one form or another. There is the guilt well spouses feel for all those unnecessary and pointless fights they had. It is the guilt felt for all the hurts inflicted that come back to haunt; all of those things said and done during the course of a marriage that spouses wish they could take back but know they can't, now they realize how unknowingly fragile their relationship was and how precious their spouse is. I guess we can never really appreciate anything until we are on the verge of losing it.

There is the guilt some spouses have when they feel that they may have done something to cause the disease, either by negligence (for example, a wife of an Alzheimer's patient who was sure that the disease was a result of her not providing healthy food for her husband) or by accident, as a husband felt when his wife bumped her head badly on the windshield during a minor accident and years later developed Alzheimer's disease. In the absence of any specific and factual "cause" we can always find one; it becomes a handy peg to hang the free floating guilt we might feel.

There is also the guilt that the parents with a disability may feel who have burdened and negatively affected their children by all of the stress that is in the family. The guilt at times seems never ending.

My guilt is sometimes expressed by wondering why I am healthy and Cari is not. How or why did I escape? I have lived the same lifestyle these 30-odd years and I am healthy and she is not. Why am I standing and she in the wheelchair?

There is also the guilt of perceived failure when

someone is hurting within the family and I have been unable to make it better. Although I know that rationally there is nothing I have done to cause the disease and the pain, and that there is nothing I can do to eliminate either the pain or the disease, I still feel the guilt of my impotence. It is a terrible feeling of powerlessness to change anything, and there is always the wonder if there might be something I can or should be doing to make things better. Guilt is a difficult emotion to cope with; it leads to resentment and I often think the anger that I feel and display are as much a function of my guilt, as of the failed expectations that I have of myself as a protector.

Guilt is corrosive in a relationship. In many marriages it is the controlling factor that keeps the well spouse involved in the relationship. The flip side of guilt is resentment because guilt is so uncomfortable a feeling and so controlling we resent that which causes this discomfort. The resentment periodically flares up in the marriage and we have arguments about "stupid" things which only lead to more feelings of guilt. Relationships with a high-guilt component invariably are unstable because of the push/pull of the guilt/resentment mechanism. I remember a sign I saw in a window during the holiday shopping season "Give the Gift that Lasts: Give Guilt." The guilt lasts, but it ultimately undermines the stability of the relationship because of the resentment that it breeds.

The well spouse often, like a careful investor, must begin to limit his or her losses. Emotionally, living with someone with chronic illness is to suffer and to experience chronic grief: this is immensely painful at times. What frequently happens, in order to limit the emotional loss, is that the shadow spouse withdraws; it hurts too much to stay intensely involved in the relationship only to experience pain. I find myself withdrawing from Cari many times as the emotions become too intense for me. Often this disengagement is expressed as a loss of feeling for her, a going through the motions sensation which feels like I am not really being present emotionally: I become detached. This engenders a great deal of guilt as I feel I should be more involved but I think it is a normal response. I think all shadow spouses must develop some self-protective mechanisms—without them it is too easy to go bankrupt emotionally. I find that after I have my emotional time out I can return to a more normal feeling of intimacy in our relationship although it is never quite the same. Our emotional relationship is always tinged with the specter of MS hanging between us.

Another feeling that is triggered by the disease is a feeling of vulnerability. There is a recognition of how fragile and tenuous our hold on life and health is. Nobody is immune from disability; it is the feeling of "There, but for the grace of God, go I." This is not so much a bad feeling as it is an uncomfortable one to give up the "cloak of invulnerability" that most of us wear in order to avoid thinking about our own intimations of mortality. This resembles very much the fear I feel that I might get ill and not be able to take care of Cari, but this fear is the existential one of the realization of how fragile and tenuous my own hold on health and life is. We are brought back to the basics by this disease and recognize that everything is just on loan to us and that the loan can be called in at any time.

The trick, I think, in dealing with feelings is to recognize that feelings just are; that I never have to be responsible for how I feel, just for how I behave.

Feelings need to be acknowledged and accepted. When that happens, the behavior can be transformed into positives rather than negatives: the anger becomes an energy to make changes; the feelings of inadequacy and confusion become the impetus to learn; the guilt becomes commitment, and the grief seems to intensify all of our feelings. The realization of our vulnerability, while uncomfortable, can also lead to very positive behaviors. For me it has led to a restructuring of priorities. I no longer waste time, and appreciate what time I have. I had never really marvelled at my ability to walk until I watched my wife stumble across a room; and she marvels repeatedly at the simple task of moving one foot in front of the other.

There is a great deal of despair in these illnesses —the feeling of helplessness and the realization that this will continue for the rest of your life; the feeling that there is no way out, that you are trapped; and always the sadness for what might have been. And yet within this despair, there are some very positive emotions. One can both love and hate intensely the other being who is so consuming. Sometimes these positive feelings are only momentary and few and far between, but these are the times that you feel tenderness and compassion for your spouse; the times you wish ardently to be able to take away some of the pain and fear.

> My heart really breaks for him. I have a lot of pity for him. Not the syrupy kind of pity. It's just that I see such a vital man really being attacked and not being able to take aspirin or to get a shot that will make him feel better. And he insists that I help him by just being there, by being supportive and not being angry with him, if he doesn't want to go to dinner or whatever. It's just that I can't have that illness with him.

There is the sustaining hope you feel in a cure or in the indication that the disease has not progressed further. There is the joy that is felt when a goal is accomplished and the pride that you feel in your own strength. We give to life what life demands of us. Chronic illness in a loved one puts a great deal of stress on us, but in the course of dealing with that stress we also find and develop those inner resources that lie latent within us all, we experience joy. Happiness, according to the poet, is a matter of having something to do, someone to love, and something to hope for. Chronic illness in a spouse can give us all of this and more. These diseases are powerful teachers.

CHAPTER 2

The Disability Marriage

Despite the marriage vow "in sickness or in health," I never really expected to, nor was I really prepared to, deal with Cari's illness—certainly not the chronic, progressive rest-of-your-life illness that is multiple sclerosis. I have yet to find a spouse who was prepared.

All marriages involve a contract.[4] The contract is comprised of a set of expectations and promises that may or may not be shared with the spouse. More often than not the contract is an implied one. The expectations we have about our marriage are based in large measure on our parents' marriage. This is the marriage we know best, having observed it from inside the family. From this information we shape our ideas about what we want from our spouse and what we are prepared to give. My parents were both quite healthy. My father died rather quickly from cancer, shortly after I was married, and Cari's parents were also quite healthy, living well past 80—her mother is still alive past 90—so neither of us had a model of spouse disability or chronic illness to work from. And like most couples we entered marriage sure it was going to last and that we would live forever; never for a minute dreaming that either of us would be disabled.

The early conflicts that couples have are usually

part of the healthy process of forging the joint contract. For most Americans, brought up on the idealized versions of marriage as portrayed on television (for example, "The Brady Bunch," "The Donna Reed Show," and so forth), conflict in marriage is to be avoided, or, when conflict does emerge, it is considered bad. Actually it is those early conflicts that ultimately strengthen the marriage by producing a clear contract. Marriages are not made in heaven, they are forged on earth and in the trenches by two people in a fair fight.

A major source of marital conflict occurs when there is continuous and chronic contractual disappointment; that is, when significant aspects of the contract are not being fulfilled over a long period of time. This happens when the expectations are not made explicit or when they are made explicit and the marital partner cannot or will not meet them. The disappointed partner may react with anger, depression, or withdrawal which in turn provokes more marital discord; such relationships begin to founder on the shoals of their mutual angers and disappointments. What a marriage counselor tries to do is to help a struggling couple make explicit their contractual demands to see if they can be made complementary; if not, the couple eventually will separate, or live very separate, unhappy lives together.

From the outside, some marriages look as if they were made in hell, but there invariably is some mutual contract satisfaction that keeps the couple in their masochistic dance. In the same vein some marriages look ideal from the outside when in reality the couple is living in a marital hell. One can never judge someone else's marriage. At heart the chemistry of a successful, healthy marriage is ineffable; in the admixture, there needs to be a mutual liking and a shared value system. There also must be some clear and open communication. At all times there must be a willingness to renegotiate the marital contract because contracts on any or all levels must be dynamic—they are constantly changing as the needs of the marital pair changes. In one sense, successful marriage is always a continuous process of accommodation.

The marriage contract is as much a state of mind as it is an actual legal document. In the course of writing this book, I have met heterosexual couples who were living together without benefit of matrimony and homosexual couples who were also as committed to each other as legally married partners. The bonds of couples are formed out of their need satisfaction and are quite independent of the legal system. Marital contract as used in this book refers to the emotional commitment of couples rather than the legalistic contract of a formal marriage ceremony.

One change that requires a vast modification of the marital contract is when a spouse has a significant illness. The specific crisis that occurs at the time of diagnosis of an illness usually pulls a family together. Short-term difficulties cause people in the family to set aside their personal agendas and rise above individual problems in order to help one another. An immediate crisis has a way of bringing out that which is most noble in many people.

The long-term chronic problem, however, is a different species. When people realize that the condition is forever, the anger, jealousies, and resentments begin to emerge, and the chronic illness can, and does, become a divisive factor in many families. Most of the more peripheral family members drift back to managing their own lives after the initial crisis subsides, leaving to the well spouse the problem of managing the chronically ill partner. More often than not, the other family members provide only marginal support after the initial crisis of the diagnosis has passed.

Cari and I were quite open with our families about the diagnosis of MS. In telling the family we were so determined to be matter of fact about it and not to let MS change our lives that we successfully dissipated any sense of crisis. In the beginning stages, it was easy because Cari was relatively symptom-free, and the slow nature of the decline has allowed all of us to gradually adjust to the illness. Our children finished their growing up and have left home. My siblings (Cari is an only child) are also matter-of-fact about her illness. My brother, sister, and mother live at a distance and we do most of our communication via telephone. While I know that they are interested and concerned they are also remote from the daily aspects of living with a spouse with MS. Our children are also very much caught up in their own lives, and have little energy or time to devote to our problems, not that there is much that they could do at this point other than to indicate their awareness and interest. The burden falls on me and Cari to manage her illness.

This has meant that our marital "contract" is constantly being renegotiated, if not formally, certainly by events as she becomes increasingly disabled and I have to assume ever increasing responsibilities within the home and within the marriage. This was not what either one of us bargained for.

In addition to being a contract, marriage is also a balancing act. We tend to marry complementary; that is, we seek in a mate that which is deficient in ourselves and we admire in others. We usually find wholeness in the couple that may not be in any one partner. Thus if one person is outgoing the other is usually inhibited, if he is a talker she is a listener; if he is an accumulator she is a thrower-outer.

Whenever we are stressed, and to be married to someone who has a chronic illness is to be stressed all the time, those qualities that are alien to us but that attracted us to our mates become flash points for our anger. In the romantic phase of the relationship the complementary characteristics are endearing but during heavy stress time they become annoying, and previously perceived strengths become weaknesses.

In our marriage, Cari is the collector and I am the thrower-outer. I don't know if that was true of us before we were married because sometimes the complementary characteristic is forced on us by the excesses of the spouse (if left to my own devises I might be a closet accumulator). I feel that because of Cari's (as I see it) inability to let go of things we would not be able to walk in the door as she has an incredible ability to clutter up a room with things and therefore I must become the disposer in the family. I feel that because of my efforts to keep things clear that the house is moderately inhabitable. We both saw what could happen in my father-in-law's house. His accumulating nature (I think this is genetic) was kept in check by his second wife. When she developed Alzheimer's disease and became disabled, he was then an accumulator unchecked. After he died and we had the unpleasant task of cleaning out their condo we found bags of materials on just about every surface in the rooms, closets stuffed to the gills, and drawers overflowing. Even though I have pointed out to Cari repeatedly what an abject lesson this was for "accumulators," it has not altered her behavior much, and the "accumulator" versus "disposer" conflict is ever present in our marriage. In actuality, this conflict keeps us in balance. Because of Cari's efforts, there is still memorabilia around and some previous discards that we have rediscovered a need for; because of my efforts there also is room to move about the house.

There are times, however, when I enter a room and see clutter and a huge ball of fury wells up in me. These are invariably times when I am most stressed or distressed about her MS and we might have a doozy of a fight about the "clutter" but the heart of the matter is my fear and anxiety and sheer fatigue in dealing with her MS. I have to recognize this in myself and acknowledge it to Cari in order to preserve our marriage and our sanity. If I do not acknowledge this from time to time our fights can lead to an increasing downward spiral into marital discord.

In my experience of working with healthy spouses of the chronically ill, it seems to me that the families who grow and prosper through the adversity of the disability are the older, longer married couples whose companionship has been tested over the years; they can take on the added stress of a disease. The others that succeed are the newly married couples who enter into the marriage knowing about the disease and have consciously made their choice openly and honestly, although nobody can know co-disability until you live with it.

Here is Karen's story of being married to a blind diabetic man. She was probably the best prepared shadow spouse I had met having lived with a diabetic father.

I was 21 and Bob was 24 when we were married. At that time he was sighted. He had been a diabetic since he was eleven years old. We both went to the same high school, but we didn't meet until we were in college. We sat next to each other in college so we started going out together and actually married before we finished college. One of the things that got us together was that we had something in common. My dad, at the age of 50, became a diabetic and my dad was a real example to me. When my dad came home from the doctor's with the regimen to follow, his diet and his insulin and so forth, he handed it to my mother and said, "This is the way we're going to cook from now on." It didn't cause that much of an uproar in our family. It was no big deal. After I met Bob and saw how he was struggling with the diabetes, I tried to help him see the more positive side.

I think it was the second date that we went on where he actually told me that he was a diabetic and I said, "So what?" He was testing me because he felt that diabetes was a negative thing. A girl had just broken up with him because he was a diabetic. After that, I started inviting him over to our house. He loved my mother's cooking. He came over quite often and we had a wonderful courtship.

Before we got married, my dad talked with his doctor and his doctor told him that diabetics have a life span of 20 years. So he sat down with me one day and said, "I just want you to know what to expect." My folks were never negative about the situation. My folks were deeply religious people. My father was a minister and he told me Bob had a life expectancy of 20 years. I said, "Dad, I would rather spend 10 good years with him than with anyone else I know. I'm willing to take that risk and I want you to let me take that risk," and he accepted it. Neither of my parents ever said anything more about it.

We got married in August and I think it was in December that he started having spots before his eyes. When he went to the doctor, it was the same month I was expecting my daughter, he found that he was losing his sight. The doctor gave him 6 months to lose it—it actually took two years. We were very upset and we did the best we could. He was still able to drive during that year that I was expecting and Helen was born. She was a delightful baby and I think she did a lot for us. At that time I was teaching; he had to change his major. He was going to be an Industrial Arts teacher. He changed his major to social studies and he finally graduated. In the meantime, when he started to go blind, his diabetes began to stabilize—usually when the eyesight begins to go, the heart and the kidneys go, too. So we were very frightened. Two other fellows that Bob was in college with, who were diabetics, were also going blind and within five years both of them were dead. So within the early years of our marriage, I really lived with that fear and so did he. Every time he bought a new suit, he'd say, "You can bury me in this." And I'd say, "Like hell I will!"

Then the adjustment to blindness on top of the diabetes was very hard. Blindness and diabetes do not go together! They work against each other because with the diabetes you need the diet and the exercise. When you are blind, it's hard to get the exercise and keep track of your diet, and it's also hard to take care of your insulin need. We've been through all those things for all these years. He finally graduated from college and he couldn't find a job. He would have been hired in one teaching position if he knew Braille. I was teaching and he was home taking care of Helen. He was learning Braille with a home teacher; it wasn't easy. It took him about 10 years to get comfortable with Braille and he was very fortunate because many diabetics do not have the sensitivity of touch to be able to do that. He did go totally blind. We found out there was a teacher education program in Boston to train people to be teachers of the blind. So we went to the school for the blind where we both were accepted for the program. Bob was still going through the adjustment and was very depressed.

Fortunately, we had two or three months of very intensive counseling which helped us both a great deal and that got us over the really tough part, but the adjustment was slow. There was a period of two weeks when Bob wouldn't talk to me. There were many days when we barely made it to counseling and we came through the counseling stronger.

During that time he was still insulin dependent; nothing has ever changed as far as his insulin dependency. He takes his shot every morning. I usually give it to him. He has to adjust to the activity of the day and if he has a cold or something, he has to watch it very carefully with a blood test. I remember one very scary time after we were first married about one month, one night he went into a severe insulin reaction and I knew what I had to do but he was so far gone into the reaction. I said to him, "Do you need sugar," and he grabbed my hand and held me so tight I didn't think he would let me go. I did get some sugar and got him out of it and I thought, "My God. What have I gotten into?" but there have only been two very severe reactions over the years.

Karen thought she was as well prepared as anyone could be, having lived with a diabetic father, but as you can see from her narrative, it is never easy. It is the day-to-dayness and the rest-of-your-lifeness that ultimately wears you down. You must constantly be prepared to change as new demands are made. Caring for someone on a short-term basis or only in a peripheral capacity is relatively easy. One can be loving and giving when you know that you can return to a "normal" life in a short while, but when you live with it constantly you are stressed to the maximum. It is also to be noted in Karen's narrative that counseling was a big help.

It is difficult to obtain any reliable statistics on the divorce rate in "disability marriages" but all researchers agree that it is high. Diabetics in the 20-to-44-year-old group have a 50% higher divorce rate than the general population, but younger and older diabetics have similar divorce rates as the general population; what is excluded from these data is how many marriages no longer have any satisfaction for the participants.

Chronic illness brings out in a marriage that which was latent and the ways in which the couple deals with the disease will be consistent with the ways in which they deal with any other stresses—only more so. Weak marriages are much more likely to crumble under the added weight of the disability, while strong marriages strengthen.

Having a spouse with a chronic disability does not necessarily lead to a divorce or an estrangement. The disability causes stress on the marital relationship by altering the marriage contract, violating expectations, and exposing weakness that might otherwise be papered over. You simply cannot "fake it" living with someone who has a chronic, progressive illness; your marriage is tested fully. With some marriages the exposed cracks are so deep that the foundation crumbles. In other marriages the stress, caused by the disability, is an occasion for working and strengthening the marriage bond, and cementing the cracks so that a stronger foundation can be put in place.

The disability marriage has several characteristics, the major one being that it is no longer a 50-50 proposition. Depending on the rate of decline and the degree of help from other family members, the shadow spouse either slowly or very rapidly assumes chores or responsibilities that the affected mate was previously responsible for. There is an ever migrating equator of marital responsibility; wives now find themselves for the first time having to balance check books and repair appliances; able-bodied husbands are suddenly doing the cooking, the family wash, and the shopping.

You can see the role reversal clearly in Alzheimer's disease and in Elizabeth's story:

About six months after the diagnosis, Al had to leave work. He was very happy when he left work; he told the doctor, "I know that I can no longer do my work, I know that they are slipping me easier work constantly, and I cannot even do that." So he went out, thank God, on long-term disability. So financially, with social security, we were able to do it. He also had the male ego thing. He was always so proud that he could support his family and now he could no longer work.

"What were we going to do?" he kept saying, and I had to convince him that he was still bringing income into the family and that he was still supporting the family. I finally got through to him but I would have to reinforce that every so often because he was devastated that he wasn't going into work.

So I became the smart person; I knew everything in his eyes. Now this is a role reversal because I always leaned on him; it was very difficult for me. We had always discussed things but my husband always made the decisions, which I agreed with. With this disease, I've had to make all the decisions.

I have to say my husband was an excellent patient while he could be and he held on for a long time. I worked across the street for many years and I was able to come home and give him his lunch when he was unable to prepare his lunch for himself. I left him on his own many times with a prayer to the Blessed Mother and with my heart beating fast. One time he put a ladder on a picnic table and fell down so I was always afraid to leave him. When I would say to him, "Would you like me to leave work and stay home with you?" he'd say, "Why would you want to? I'm fine." And when the time came when I did have to say, "You must have me with you," he accepted it perfectly. We lived for the next few years with me at his side constantly.

He took himself off the road. One day he just said, "I will not drive any longer." I was thankful for that because I was sitting next to him very ready to grab the wheel and step on the brake. I always tried to let him hold his human dignity as best I could, and tried not to take things away from him.

Then he began to get into deep trouble. He wasn't sleeping properly and he would get up from a night and wander and I would say, "Al, Al, please stay in bed; I need my sleep and you need yours." And maybe I would have to put him back in several times and he would know he was doing this. He would say, "I know but I can't help it." I finally had to sleep on a sofa in another room with the door open so I could hear. Sleep is a strange word for it because you really didn't sleep. You rested out of exhaustion but I made sure I could hear. I must have slept there for eight months.

And I saw him getting worse. He would see things that I didn't see and I'd say, "Oh, you're talking nonsense. There's nobody there." We'd go for a ride, he liked to ride, and he'd see things that weren't there and they were hallucinations only I didn't realize that's what it was. I just passed it off "Oh, you're talking foolish."

From there it was hell, watching him deteriorate was like pieces from a broom being pulled right out of him. Every bit of his human dignity; every bit of the man. Every bit. It was hell. He is now incontinent. He was a very meticulous man all the years of our married life. I never had to pick up after him.

The savior now is that he is no longer aware. While he was aware, there was a hell within a hell because he knew he could no longer remember. He would struggle, and to watch him struggle to walk over and try to get a drink of water and be incapable of it. It was just overwhelming for him and for me. He just got worse and worse. He got so bad at home. He could take none of the outside world. None. My grandchild would stand and do nothing and he would agitate; his whole body would shake. He couldn't take anything. We were sending him to day care; the woman at day care described him as a bomb about to go off. From this mild-mannered man, to this completely degenerated mind is horrendous.

The role reversal is a difficult issue in all disability marriages but it seems particularly more difficult for the wives in a more traditional marriage as Elizabeth's marriage appears to be. In these traditional marriages, the woman is generally in a more dependent position both financially and emotionally than the husband. The financial prospects of her becoming the principal bread winner in the family are often overwhelming and sometimes, more cogently, the loss of respect for her husband's mental and physical capabilities are often devastating. Elizabeth has to make a profound adjustment. Unlike the suddenly widowed, she has to do it while her husband is alive and in many respects this makes the adjustment more difficult. There is always the judgement to be made as to when to step in and take over the function that the spouse previously had: as Elizabeth had to do with her husband's driving. Sometimes this shifting of family functions is done subtly and the shadow spouse awakes to the realization that he or she is exhausted by living at home. I have yet to meet the well spouse of an Alzheimer's patient who did not look at least ten years older than their stated age. I also found several who were so exhausted that they needed to be hospitalized.

In a successful non-disability marriage, the giving and getting generally work out equitably over the long haul. In cases where a spouse is temporarily disabled or absent, the other spouse can fill in comfortably for a period of time when they recognize that their partner is temporarily needy and is not capable of giving. They are secure in the belief that things will get better. But the spouse in a disability marriage knows that his/her partner is never going to be able to do more than they are currently doing and probably will be able to do even less in the future. The shifting balance of responsibility is never stable with chronic illness—there is always progression, and with progression there is more shifting of the load; it is like a child's seesaw in which the healthy end is continuously moving closer to the ground and the marital responsibilities, which had started out in the middle, are slowly shifting to the healthy spouse's end.

In my marriage I have been slowly assuming more and more responsibilities for the running of the house. I am essentially doing all the shopping and a great deal of the cooking. I was trying to keep up with the housework and finding it impossible to do; I finally have agreed to hire a cleaning service and I now think that is the best money we could have spent. It has taken a great deal of the burden off of me and I am beginning to see how necessary it is for me to purchase services where I can and also to ask for help from friends, family, and neighbors. There is no way I can do this entirely on my own and I have come to recognize this.

Another common theme running through disability marriages is the issue of increasing dependency; with increasing dependency comes the need to control the other. If you feel that you cannot survive on your own then you need to control those around you so that they can be there to satisfy your needs. Very often the dependency manifests itself as a heightened concern about the well spouse's health and safety. Although Cari always supports my leaving on a trip, she also is concerned about my welfare. When I was recently invited to take a (not commercial) plane ride by a friend she answered empathetically "no" for me. (Cari claims this has nothing to do with her MS.) When I am already feeling burdened, the reminder to take extra care only sparks a fight because now I feel that I am also responsible for her fear and anxiety. It is hard enough coping with the full freight of my own fears; I don't want or need to carry her's too.

Jack, whose wife has arthritis feels much the same way:

> I have found I cannot run my life that way. I have to live everyday as I see it. I cannot worry about tomorrow. And that causes a conflict because she thinks that I do things that are not appropriate, and by appropriate she means to the situation we find ourselves in because of the disease that she could not step in and survive as a single parent. I think she thinks of herself as being more dependent than she re-

ally is. I think she overreacts to it. She isn't as dependent as she thinks she is.

Couples need to get to the core issues of the dependency and recognize it for what it is: a natural concomitant of chronic, progressive illness. In a disability marriage the well spouses have an obligation to maintain their health a bit more because they have used up their safety margins as a family and do not have the fail-safe, dual system that exists in most other families. There is the fear I feel when I pick my way across the ice and think if I fell and broke my leg what would happen to us. But like Jack I also recognize I cannot live in constant fear limiting my choices. If I fell and injured myself, somehow we would manage; we must.

With the change in responsibilities comes a change in the power balance in the marriage. It is hard to maintain equality or the feelings of equality when one spouse is becoming increasingly dependent on the other. Cari's increasing dependency on me leaves her less inclined to assert herself as an equal partner in our marriage. She seems much more inclined to do what I want to do in order to please me and not anger me. She sometimes has said that she doesn't have the power to leave and yet would not be surprised if I might choose to do so. As I see it, her way of re-establishing some dominance in our relationship is to become very critical of the domestic tasks that I have had to assume because of her increasing disability. For example, I never seem to be able to make the bed properly or to fold the laundry to her satisfaction. In fact, there are times when it seems I can do nothing right. The message she is trying to send me is that I still need her, unfortunately I don't always hear that, and I more often than not respond with anger or annoyance. I think this also may be a matter of her losing control of her body and therefore needing to control others. It is only when I stop and think about what is going on that I can be more accepting of her criticism.

Also with dependency comes increased anger of the loss of control of her life. This has been, for example, a very hard winter with a great deal of snow and ice, so much so that Cari has not been able to leave the house for over two months. And although she often doesn't realize it or mean it, there are days that the confinement and loss of control gets the best of her and, since I am the handiest target, I get some of the displaced anger. Cari is sensitive about inflicting pain on others, but there are times she can contain her anger no longer and those are the days that I feel buried under an avalanche of complaints and orders. I do recognize that if our positions were reversed I would be much more abusive than she ever is, because most of the time she is an "up" person. I often tell her that I have put in her application for sainthood and she just might become the first Jewish Saint!

For my part I have to be careful to respect her personhood and, although the marriage is no longer equal in many ways, there are still many areas in which she remains a peer. I don't always see this and I will occasionally not consider her needs as I blunder ahead doing what I want to do. It is dangerous for me to think that, because I am the able-bodied one, I can have it all my way. We get into trouble when I do this. In many ways having a chronically ill spouse seems like having a dependent child with the growth process reversed.

Sometimes the power struggle works out differently, with the able-bodied spouse bending over backwards to the point of self abnegation, in order to maintain the chronically ill spouse's self-esteem. Here is Karen, again, co-disabled by diabetes:

> The diabetes has changed my life. I know that I was perfectly capable of going on and getting my doctorate but I determined early on that if we were going to make this marriage work that Bob was going to come first and that's the way it's always been. I was tempted to go on many times. I know what I can handle. Every once in a while Bob says to me, "Why don't you apply here or there?" and I tell him, how can I when he comes home every night with so much work that I have to help him with. We are still putting in so many hours working that it stopped what I could have done. I am also content because I can see what he is doing so I can live with it. I sometimes feel like I am living a double life. I have my professional life in which I am the only teacher of the visually impaired in my school system and I have that satisfaction where I can work and tell teachers what they should do with a child and I have a lot of professional recognition. And I have a great deal of freedom. At home with Bob I am the "little woman." Bob is the head of the house and when I come home I say, "What do we do next?" and I think to myself am I really lowering myself to do this and then I think, no I'm doing it to maintain the leadership qualities that he needs in his job. I have my outlet in sewing. When things go bad, I go and sew.

In another life, Karen might have been more overtly assertive of her own needs. In dementia, the power shift is most obvious, because the able spouse is increasingly assuming an adult role to the child-like spouse. In other diseases, it is more subtle but present nonetheless. Dominance/dependency issues run through all disability marriages; and almost all marital disputes that are not about contract disappointment are about control issues.

Most chronic illness is variable and it is so easy for the well spouse to be insensitive. Jack, the husband of Ann, who has arthritis:

I think the most difficult thing for me is probably being a
good husband and friend sometimes because you tend to forget that your wife is different than other people. That is,
that emotionally she will go through a lot of peaks and val-
leys that other people won't go through. Some days she will
just get terribly down and other days everything is fine but I
don't know what those days are. Yet it takes you maybe two
hours to say, "Oh, maybe this isn't a great day," and sometimes you may even think it's you that is not right. That is
probably one of the most difficult things to experience because my wife is also my best friend and you want to do a lot
of things together and she might not be up to doing it. And
you get disappointed and you think more about yourself
than you think about her. It's difficult to get through all of
that because there are days when she thinks nothing is
right. It's the despair that comes out of having to deal with
pain on a daily basis.

In the disability marriage, the disease can, and
often does, become the central focus of the marriage.
Increasing time and energy that used to be devoted to
maintaining the marriage are consumed by the disease
or, more specifically, by reactions to the demands of the
disease. My wife has commented that all of her energy
is devoted to getting from point A to point B, so that at
times she doesn't have much left over to think about
anything else. Illness sometimes demands an intense
self-absorption that can become characteristic of a seriously ill person. This self-absorption sometimes
defeats Cari's efforts to feel like something other than
a rolling (I used to say walking) illness. There are
many times when I also feel as if she is lost to multiple
sclerosis. It sometimes feels to me that the more I take
over the tasks she needs me to do, the more she and
the disease take control of me. My life, at times, seems
to become a steady accumulation of meeting another
person's needs and I wonder when I ceased becoming a
husband and instead became a caretaker.

One of the ways Cari and I have learned to deal with what, at times, seems to me to be the incessant demands on my time is that now when I choose to, I can declare a moratorium. I will tell her that for the next two hours, she cannot ask me to do anything; in fact, I tell her she cannot talk to me. All moratoria, though, are always followed by a period in which I will do anything she wishes, no questions asked. This simple rule has maintained my sanity, preserved Cari's dignity, and it gives us both some measure of control over our lives.

Another characteristic of the disability marriage is that an increasing amount of a couple's social life is with people who have a similar disability. It becomes so much easier for us to socialize with fellow "MSers." They understand instantly and intuitively what our needs are and what we are going through. Frequently, they have made the necessary environmental compensations that make living and getting around easier for the disabled. There is a disabled community that is immensely helpful and sharing. The down side is that it is hard to find friends whom you would have liked and been interested in anyway were it not for the disability tie, because there is such a limited pool of people to select from. In many disability relationships or friendships, there is not much left to the relationships once you strip away the commonality of the disease.

One of the major roles of a spouse in a working marriage is as a source of emotional support. A spouse is the most likely person to provide needed help when you are troubled. As the spouse becomes more disabled and more disease-dominated, he or she is unable to provide emotional support to the well spouse. In fact, the person can be so emotionally needy that the healthy spouse often must seek support outside of the marriage. This is especially true of the dementing diseases. Our parents are our link to the past and our children are our link to the future; our spouse gives us the present. With the loss of a viable spouse there is a deep loss of that shared present. At times, if I am not careful, I feel as if my life with a spouse who has a chronic, progressive illness is narrowing down to a tight circle of lonely misery.

When I am in public with my wife, we stand out in a crowd; we are no longer like everyone else. There are scenes etched in my mind like a vivid photograph never to fade. I can remember the first time Cari used a wheelchair in an airport and I wheeled her to an area to the side of the departure gate. There was also another couple with a wife standing by her husband's wheelchair. As the wife and I exchanged glances over the backs of chairs, I realized at a gut level that I was no longer like everybody else. I had just joined a new fraternity and the other shadow spouse seemed to be welcoming me to the club—a club neither one of us wanted to join. We never said anything to each other but there seemed to be an acknowledgement, and perhaps it was for me the first time that I emotionally acknowledged to myself that I had "MS too" and for this reason, that scene is burned into my memory with a level of clarity I have almost never known.

The wife of a man with MS commented, "When we go to a restaurant and my husband has to go to the bathroom, he staggers across the room. He will not use a cane or wheelchair and I know that everyone watching him is sure he is drunk. I cringe."

The loss of anonymity is a feeling akin to embarrassment or even guilt. There is a vague feeling that you have done something wrong to merit the looks you get in public places. I always feel that I have to explain to the watchers that she has multiple sclerosis and neither she nor I did anything to deserve this. The loss of anonymity very often seems to allow people to ask thoughtless questions and to make, at times, very insensitive comments. My wife can hardly go out in her wheelchair without being "God-Blessed" right and left. Adults often speak loudly to her as though she can't hear or talk to me over her head as though she can not understand. Children are often a delight in their naive interest and willingness to help; the adults with their stares and comments are often boorish. I think I understand now that the disabled, particularly ones like Cari in a wheelchair, remind everyone of their own vulnerability—the "There, but for the grace of God, go I" syndrome, and that causes most people to feel uncomfortable. Most people don't know what to do around the disabled and there is a great deal of awkwardness and discomfort.

How easy it used to be when I could say to my wife, "Let's go to the movies," and we would go. (That was after the children were grown sufficiently so that we did not have to get babysitters!) Now going someplace involves considerable amounts of planning. We have to calculate how accessible a place is and whether or not they can accommodate our needs. Places we go now need to be scouted for bathroom accessibility, vehicle accessibility, and how many steps are involved; we can no longer spontaneously decide to go anywhere. This is true for all the illnesses; there is always a restriction on the freedom of movement. The rule of thumb with someone who is in a wheelchair is that things will take three times as long. As I watch Cari shower and dress in the morning or cook, doing all the so-called affairs of daily living, I am struck at how much time and effort is involved; her morning ablutions take at least one hour. Going any place with her is a similar experience. Until she can get herself together and I can get her into the van, the better part of an hour has been lost. I know I have to allow maximum time and not try to get very much done on a given day; we have to pick our excursions carefully.

Whenever we go out (a big date for us is the mall for lunch and shopping) the first place Cari heads for is the ladies room. I stand outside waiting patiently or impatiently as the case may be. I am composing material for my next book, which according to family legend is, "What to do while your wife is in the ladies room." Actually I am praying fervently that she does not get into trouble and I might have to go in and help her. I was badly scarred this past summer when we went to a wedding at a country club and the toilets were not handicapped accessible. (I guess they did not cater to golfers with any handicaps.) When Cari had to use the facilities I had to go with her and I found myself in the ladies room frantically helping Cari adjust her clothing, surrounded by a group of women impatiently waiting to use the toilets. (A few bold ones went ahead and used the stall but no one offered to help.) I could not think of a place or a situation that I would rather be in less and so each time Cari goes into a public restroom I get immensely religious and pray that she will be able to take care of herself.

Sometimes this toilet thing goes from the sublime to the ridiculous, worthy of a *Far Side* cartoon. Recently, in going to see a play, Cari took with her a toilet insert that elevates the level of the toilet and makes it easier for her to get off and on the seat. She carried it in a plastic trash bag in the basket of her wheelchair. As I watched the play I wondered what the other people would think if they knew what was in that bag. After a while I did not care because Cari said it worked like a charm and it saved me from having to mount a rescue mission.

Most of us like to think that we have an unlimited range of choices to be who or what we would like to be. Progressive disability is often like a noose slowly tightening around life's options, restricting choices and limiting opportunities. (Other doors open but that is not always seen.) The wife of a man with MS feels anger and resentment because her children had finally left home and she was ready to go back to school and now "the MS is restricting me at a time when I am just ready to reach out and expand."

I feel restrictions on my mobility in terms of seeking new opportunities and facing the trauma of moving and making changes. Cari says I am putting these restrictions on myself and that it's not a function of her MS. She is probably right. The danger is that I allow her multiple sclerosis to become an excuse for me. It is always hard to distinguish between internal constraints and external restraints. There are many things we can do and I choose not to do them because of the increased hassle required. After reading an article about some person in a wheelchair who traveled to an exotic place, Cari will comment that we could go too. She invariably admires the person in the chair while I (not in one of my better moments) comment that all she did was sit and everybody else did the work. Cari is right we could go if we chose to and I recognize that the choice is always there. Of course I must also suffer the consequences of my choices; we are defined in life by the choices we make. And at this point in my life I prefer the less stressful living in our adapted home to the uncertainties and stress of travel.

As I mentioned previously, the biggest loss in chronic, progressive disability is the loss of the expected future. Cari and I had many plans, most of which assumed a vigorous and mobile middle age for both of us. These dreams have to be modified or cannot even be formulated because the future is shrouded in such uncertainty. It feels like there is no foundation to the future; it is built on shifting sands that are always undermining any "structure" we might build. No one's future is certain, but with progressive disability the uncertainty is more apparent.

Probably the hardest thing for us at this time is to see a middle-aged couple in the midst of some vigorous activity. For example, what brought the tears stinging to our eyes was watching a couple on a beach walking with their dog, so obviously enjoying good health and each other. It is not so much that we envy them, as that, in watching them, we recognize anew our loss and grieve for it. Every so often, when we least expect it, the gaping chasm of the loss becomes apparent and we must allow ourselves the time and place to grieve—then pick ourselves up and go on. It's not the big losses we stumble over, it's the little ones like not being able to go for a walk on a lovely autumn evening or being unable to show my wife the newest addition to the garden.

In many of the diseases described in this book, the disabled spouse will have impaired sexual functioning: many men with multiple sclerosis or diabetes are impotent; woman may experience a loss of genital sensation. One shadow spouse was totally turned off sexually by his wife's need to use a catheter, and it is difficult at times to see a severely disabled person as sexually desirable. It's hard to make love with someone who is wearing diapers. For arthritic people, all movement involves pain, and sex with a demented partner can be hazardous at best. Healthy spouses are generally going to have to live with some loss of sexual stimulation, and all will have to modify their sexual expectations. In working with shadow spouses, the issue of sex, or the lack thereof, emerges fairly quickly. I am struck at the variety of solutions couples can find, and I have come to the conclusion that what happens in the privacy of the bedroom, as long as there is consent between the couples, is okay.

Couples in which sexual congress is difficult and/or not possible must find the intimacy of closeness and stroking as a substitute for intercourse. There really is no substitute for intimacy in our lives but we can find release and substitutes for our sexuality.

Affairs for well spouses are not uncommon, although, because of the energy demands and time constraints imposed by living with a chronically ill spouse, it is very difficult, if not impossible, to find the time and space to have an extramarital affair. Most "affairs" are conducted in the imagination. For me, knowing that being discovered having an extramarital affair would devastate Cari restrains me—although I understand fully the temptation. Any momentary pleasure I might have with another woman is so far out-weighed by the possibility of the pain it would inflict, that having an actual affair is not an issue for me.

So why do I stay? That is a question I ponder daily. Aside from the obvious answer that I love my wife and care for her greatly, I know beyond a shadow of a doubt that if our positions were reversed and I was the one with the chronic illness (one becomes acutely aware of one's own vulnerability with illness in the family), my wife would stay the course. I also know that I could no longer live with myself if I "bugged out" when the going got tough. For me the question has no longer become whether or not I leave, but whether or not I will do the job that needs to be done.

The other aspect is that, despite the strain and pain in the disability, it is not all terrible—there are many positives in the situation. Despite the anger and despair that I have detailed, Cari and I are much closer as a result of the illness. I daily admire her courage and fortitude. She makes it much easier for me to stay as she refuses to quit ("What other course do I have?" she frequently says). As long as I feel that she is doing all she can to minimize the disability (which she is doing fully) and that she hasn't quit, I am able to get sustenance within my marriage and staying the course is relatively easy.

Some people float along the surface of their marriage never having come to grips with themselves or with each other. In a disability marriage that endures, you are tested fully; it demands change and compromise daily. It means finding the ability to endure, and the strength and courage to do what needs to be done. It means constantly grieving for the person you knew and accepting the person who is there. It means trying to get what you want and need, and learning to settle for what you have. It requires caring and commitment. It means, finally, finding within yourself the happiness and strength no other person can ever give you. The challenge to the shadow spouse is to make this happiness out of what is potentially a tragic situation; you are tested to the fullest.

CHAPTER 3

Children of Disability

Parents are the axis around which a family rotates. Parents, in a family that functions well, maintain an executive authority and dole out responsibilities to their children. The process of growing up is a matter of the child continually pushing against parental authority. Parents must give ground grudgingly until the child achieves adulthood. The need to view one's parents as strong, intelligent, and competent is a childhood illusion that is difficult to alter at any age. It is hard to know when childhood ends; we have no real markers. My brother has commented that the time he was most frightened while growing up was when he talked about a family problem and our parents actually listened to him.

Adolescents are normally granted a moratorium or postponement period during which the identity of childhood gradually merges with that of adulthood. Eventually the adolescent must give up this moratorium to assume adult responsibility. Adolescence is a cultural and social event. The biology is clear; one moment you are a child and the next minute you are capable of having children. Adolescence is a luxury that society can afford only when it is affluent. In marginal societies, the adolescent joins the work force in order to contribute to the society as soon as possible, and in poor families, within an affluent society, the adolescent is often called upon to assume adult responsibilities sooner than their better-off counterparts. My father, for example, the son of immigrant parents, left school after the eighth grade to join the workforce to become an important contributor to the family. He never had an adolescence and could not cope very well with mine (I don't know many parents who can) and we had a stormy relationship until shortly before his death.

Probably the best indication of when someone has arrived at adulthood is the willingness to see one's parents as fellow adults struggling with the very human problems of making the most of their lives. There is a predictable life crisis of adulthood that occurs when we realize that we are more capable than our parents. This is not the adolescent experience that Mark Twain described when he quipped, "When I was 15, I thought my father was the stupidest person alive. At 19, I was surprised at how much he had learned in four short years."

There does come that time for all of us, usually in our adulthood, when we realize that we really do know more than our parents. There is a role reversal that occurs and we then begin to parent our parents. This realization usually leaves us feeling very frightened and alone because we may experience for the first time, our existential aloneness and recognize that there is nobody to protect us. For most of us, the realization of our dominion over our parents usually occurs over time, fueled by many small incidents that reflect our parents' increasing incompetence.

For adolescent children of parents with disability, the moratorium phase is shortened or sometimes even nonexistent as they become "parentified" into the family and are forced to assume adult responsibilities much sooner than their peers. For these children, the normal crisis of adulthood is accelerated. They have to deal with parental incompetence at a much earlier age than they might be developmentally ready for. This can be quite frightening to self-absorbed adolescents who ordinarily see parents as unwanted intrusions on their autonomy or merely as providers for their sustenance, but rarely as people. To have to suddenly look at your father as someone who can no longer be a provider and as a person who is hurting and is fearful and who may now be dependent on you is quite frightening. From the beginning, Cari and I were determined not to burden our children with the MS. At the time of the diagnosis our two oldest children were adolescents and the third about to enter adolescence.

In preparation for writing the draft of the book I asked my oldest child, Alison to write me her views of her mother's MS. For me this was an eye-opener as I never realized the depth of her pain (perhaps I could not acknowledge it) and I can hardly read her version of our family's coping with her mother's MS without tears coming to my eyes. Here then is our family—warts and all—as seen by my oldest daughter.

> I remember my mother's step on the stairs: light, quick, determined. She must have gone up and down those stairs a hundred times a day when I was growing up, carrying loads of laundry, bathing us, chasing us back upstairs at bedtime. I remember my mother constantly in motion. She talked on the phone, made dinner, and refereed our fights simultaneously, like one of those Indian goddesses with six arms. She made casseroles and froze them and put them in the oven on self-time; she got four kids off to two or three different schools and herself off to work by 7:45 A.M.; she went up and down the block collecting for the Heart Fund, she stood on the town green for Amnesty International, she went, she went, she went.

People used to say "I don't know how your mother does it," on a regular basis and shake their heads. She made regular mothers look a little slow, a little soft. My mother walked everywhere—she didn't learn to drive until she was forty and I was sixteen. She'd fly to the supermarket a half mile away, pushing a baby stroller or carriage at a furious clip, and return just as briskly, laden with groceries, with two or three of us trotting along behind her.

She was "Wonder Woman" in her own words, and in the eyes of many other people. I admired her but I also felt isolated from her by her constant activity. She was strong-willed, wiry, and driven; I was dreamy and stubborn. Often our relationship felt like a collision between the irresistible force and the immovable object.

When I found out she had MS, I was eighteen. I had just returned from a three-month backpacking trip in Europe and was about to move out of my family's house to my first real job and my first apartment. I don't remember the words she used to tell me, but I'm sure she tried to minimize the impact of what MS meant. After all, her symptoms at the time were barely noticeable. She was still running two miles a day. I remember going down to the basement to cry and her coming after me. In an awkward attempt to comfort me she said, "Don't worry honey, it isn't hereditary." I felt like I couldn't even mourn properly what was going on with her; it wasn't my right. It was her problem and she was taking it on the chin—so was my father as far as I could see. We never cried together about it, never discussed our fears. Everyone was coping, that was my family's way.

Despite my parents' very good intentions to make this as easy on us as possible, I grieved alone and was scared alone, and I think that is also true of the other children in the family, although I don't know because we hardly ever talk about it. Before the MS, I was already the family member who cried most openly and expressed sadness and despair most readily. I felt sad and desperate about this too, but I didn't feel like I had a right to those feelings—it wasn't my disease. And there had always been such a gulf between my mother and me that I didn't feel as though I even had a right to feel bad for her. We didn't speak the same language, emotionally; what concerned her about the MS—the stigma, at first, that no one should know—and the loss of her ability to be in constant motion—were not the things that hurt or scared me.

Even as I type this, I can hear my mother's voice in my ear correcting my English usage "The MS didn't hurt you—you hurt yourself with the MS" "The MS didn't scare you—you scared yourself with the MS." Ever since she took an EST training, she has insisted on taking total responsibility for her feelings, and she corrects other people's grammar until their syntax reflects that they are taking responsiblity for their feelings too.

At first, my mother didn't even want us to tell our friends. This was *her* information, about *her* life. She is a private person, and was even more so then. I disregarded her wishes. I told my best friend, and I told my boyfriend at the time. I needed to share the information with people, even if I couldn't make sense of it properly myself.

At the time my mother was diagnosed I only had a shadowy notion of what MS really was. She explained the medical things that were happening, the myelin sheath, the nervous system, in great detail. What I didn't get, what none of us knew at the time, was what it would be like to watch her slowly, over the years, lose mobility, bladder control, to watch her head shake with palsy, to watch her inch her way precariously across a room clinging to the door-frames and just make it onto the sofa,—to watch, to watch, and not be able to do anything to stop it, or make it easier, and not to know when there would be an end to what we would have to watch. I have gone through so many emotional stances toward her MS over the years, it's hard now, after seventeen years of living with the diagnosis, to remember them all. I think at first there was the shock, that something could actually be wrong with Mom—I don't remember her ever staying in bed with a cold when I was a kid, I don't remember her ever being sick. Then here was my confusion about how calamitous it felt to me and how stoically my parents were taking it. Later, I was relieved to go along with my parents' denial and coping because that meant I could get on with my life, get on with being eighteen and not worry too much about them.

Still later, as her symptoms progressed and became

more apparent, there was grief, and fear, which would get buried and pop up over and over again. Telling new people in my life about it was illuminating. I remember mentioning casually to a housemate that my mother had MS. He turned white and his eyes filled with tears. By then the information was normal to me. I was 24, she had had MS for six years, we were all just fine. Seeing his reaction was a clue to what other emotions we could be having.

I don't think the real conscious grieving really started for me until my late twenties, as her walking became more and more precarious, and the illusion of her being able to maintain a really physically active lifestyle began to wear thin for both my parents. At the time, I was having a hard struggle with a lot of depression. I don't blame that on the MS—I think it came from other things. But on a bad day, seeing my mother try to stumble from room to room and lose ground all the time just increased my sense of despair.

She held on tight all the way, refusing to have a railing installed on the stair to the basement to make her trips to the laundry easier, resisting every modification to the house or car until the last possible moment. The rest of the family had to stand by and watch, sometimes holding our breath, as she struggled to place a heavy dish on the table, or grabbed onto a door frame or chair back just in time to keep from falling.

I felt torn; on the one hand I supported her right to make her own decisions and choices. On the other hand, it made for a lot of tension. It's hard to stand by when you're afraid someone will fall.

My father would leave on business trips and ask us kids confidentially to "check in on Mom." We'd go over there and she'd ask us sarcastically if we'd come to "babysit" her. She's let us know that she didn't need that kind of attention. Conflicting messages came at us from both sides. It was not a comfortable situation. No one knew what the rules were; should she stay alone? Can she? If we don't let her, are we being patronizing and insensitive? If we do and she falls and can't get to a phone, are we being neglectful? We didn't always have the grace of being able to do what was needed without kicking up any insecurities.

My mother didn't want to be identified as "the patient,"

"the weak one." She hated to admit she needed help. She resisted the label "disease." I remember going with her to a weekend workshop led by a famous rabbi. At one point he called for a "healing circle." Anyone who wanted healing from any kind of physical or emotional ailment could get into the circle and receive healing. By this time my mother was using a cane and had a lot of difficulty getting around. Other people whose problems, whatever they were, were much less visible, crowded into the circle. Several people looked at her expectantly. My mother sat firmly on the sidelines looking around with a bemused expression, as if to say, "Who me?"

I think it was considered shameful in my family to have a problem. My parents would both prefer to give rather than to receive. They also like to have the answers and to be in control of situations. MS is something that we can't control and have no answers for. We all agree it's a challenge, on a physical, emotional and spiritual level. My family has coped by modifying but not really changing their basic control-oriented approach to life. I very much wanted my mother to transform at another level. I thought if the MS forced her to slow down, then she might also soften and deepen and we could become closer. I wanted the MS to change her into the mother I had needed her to be when I was little; I wanted her to become someone I could talk to. I didn't give a damn about whether her legs worked or not. But of course, she cared, and cares very much about how her legs work. They're her legs. I'm the one who has had to let go of my agenda.

At one point, not too long after her diagnosis, I remember coming upon her sitting in the living room just listening to the birds singing. It seemed like she was changing. And she really has; it's just been gradually, on her own terms, as it should be. When I was growing up I don't remember her ever having any close women friends. She was too busy and she didn't trust people enough to let them in. For the last few years a group of women from her Temple have been coming by the house to do physical therapy with her. She is now rich in friends and very beloved in the community. That's a huge, significant change; although the MS has circumscribed her life, friendships have opened it up. There's no balance sheet that you can measure the gains and losses on.

It seems like there's been a back and forth seesaw kind of growth for all of us. I see my mother sometimes letting go of a few compulsions. Sometimes when we talk on the phone she doesn't correct my syntax and we have real contact. Other times, the compulsions and the constant activity are back, although they're now confined to the radius of her wheelchair. Those are the times I feel I can't get close to her. Sometimes I am able to let go of my old anger at her and just love her as she is and feel tremendous compassion and even empathy for her—it's not my legs, but I do have an imagination and I know what it means to feel frustrated, powerless, and scared. Other times I get angry and disappointed and hurt with her all over again.

For the last four years I've lived in California. When I first moved out here I thought I'd die of guilt and grief. I didn't realize how tied to my family I was. My dad had instilled in us that "Blood is thicker than water," and "The apple doesn't fall far from the tree." This apple rolled a long way. I felt terrible about inflicting another loss on my parents at a time when they were already losing so much. I felt bad about my brothers and sisters taking up the slack of the extra work that my folks need. At the same time I needed to go and it's been a good move for me. My mother encouraged me. She has tried never to cling, never to smother or hold me back. I don't know if I would have the courage she has had, not only with the MS, but with other challenges in her life.

Having this distance has helped me gain more compassion and perspective on my parents. Most of the time I'm happy living here and then there are odd moments when it hits me that I'm so far away from the family. The hardest moments for me have been the times when my mother has been in the hospital. I can't visit her or do anything. The year that she made the transition into being in a wheelchair fulltime was hard for me. All my life I'd badgered her to talk to me about her feelings. Now she was saying, "I can't believe I won't walk again. I can't believe I'll be sitting in this chair for the rest of my life." Or she'd talk about feeling sad or scared. It was what I'd asked for, but it was hard for me to receive the gift of her honest feelings. I'd hang up the phone and cry and cry. I couldn't believe anything could hurt that much. At the same time I did feel that we were sharing the pain a little and there was comfort in that time for me.

Once I likened MS to a twenty-year car crash. It's like this slow-motion disaster movie where you get to watch every frame of seeing someone's nervous system get destroyed. One way to cope is to stay focused on the frame you're watching and not play back the older frames or leap into the future. Another is to just let the pain in, and let it move through you. If I can cry really hard and just acknowledge that I'm grieving and I have a right to, then it moves and I can go on to the next moment.

The older I get the more I love my parents as people and the more I appreciate them for how they've been with me, and how well they've always tried to live their lives. They are amazing people. I don't know how to say it without sounding corny. My father has listened, loved, been there for all of us. He has taken on most of the burden, and continues to be the main nurturer of the family. I honestly don't know how I would get through it if something happened to him. I think I have a bargain going with God that nothing more bad can happen in my family because of Mom's MS, but I know there are no guarantees.

My mother hates to be called courageous, inspiring, brave—but she is all those things. She continues to be interested in other people, to find ways to engage with life, to take part in the larger community. Her unpaid vocation in life has been to work for social welfare and justice. Her smile is luminous. People stop and hug her on the street and she doesn't know what to think—she's afraid it's just because she's in a wheelchair, that they're making a fuss over her, but it's because her spirit shines very brightly, especially in the public arena where she doesn't have the same pressures on her that she's had in the family.

I'm not as close to my siblings as I am to my friends, but I appreciate them. We've been given different roles in the family; my sister has been labelled the practical, efficient one. She doesn't like the label, but she's very responsible, and has taken on a lot of the work. My oldest brother has also taken on a lot, again practical, important things like shovelling the walk or making sure the garbage cans get put out when my father travels on business. When we lived closer,

my husband and I often did airport duty—I was also as-
signed the role of the therapist to the grandparents, a job
that was bad for me. I wouldn't like to say that the MS has
brought my family together, because I don't believe that's
true, but we do share a common reality that's very big and
puts smaller things into perspective. I'm very grateful for
my siblings and their partners because they are there and I
don't feel as guilty about what I'm doing for my parents. At
some later date, in some other way, it may become my turn;
or I may find some other way to contribute to the family welfare.

I probably have a greater sense of my parents' mortality
than most people with 59-year-old parents have. I also have
a great sense of the fragility of my own health and mobility.
I don't take movement for granted. Every time I go to the Y,
run down the stairs and jump in the pool, I notice. I get
down on my hands and knees to play with a child, I dance, I
walk in the mountains, I appreciate it. I am somewhat
haunted by a fear that I will get MS. If my hands or my feet
fall asleep when I'm in bed, I'm sure it's a symptom. I worry
about being too tired. My acupuncturist tries to reassure me
that he'll make sure I won't get it. I have no faith in Western
medicine—they haven't done much for my mother except
give her treatments that have bad side effects and unknown
long-range dangers like steroids.

Life isn't fair—everyone wants a long healthy happy life
for themselves and their families, but death and suffering and
disease are part of the whole. They just are. Having a parent
with MS isn't what makes my life hard; it's my own strug-
gles to come to terms with being human that challenge me.

My oldest son, who is an Engineer deflects all of
my questions about how his mother's MS has affected
him with a shrug. It has always been hard to get him
to talk about his feelings, yet he is the one, as Alison
has commented, who will call to check that we are
okay in face of a snow storm or other natural calam-
ity. He also demonstrates his caring by being our general handyman and arrives at our house prepared to
do all the small chores my ineptness have left undone.

Our daughter Emily feels that her mother's MS affected her during adolescence by preventing her from rebelling. She felt she had to be good because she did not want to upset us. To my dismay, she is newly married and feels that she must increase her distance from us as she does not want to be sucked into a caretaker role, one that she feels she has often played out in the family.

My youngest son feels guilt that somehow he caused the MS by being born. He had read somewhere that MS was exacerbated by hormonal changes and he knew that his mother's MS was tentatively diagnosed right before his conception. I remember him as a pre-adolescent saying that he wanted to be a scientist and cure MS. He is currently getting his doctorate in neurobiology and perhaps someday he will.

There is very little information in the literature on specifically how children of disability fare. Roy,[9] in a careful review of the literature of children of disabled concluded "How much attention should the clinician pay to the children of chronically ill parents? Common sense suggests a great deal but research evidence remains equivocal." It seems to me in my experience of interviewing families and working with them professionally, that children can go either one of two ways: they become parentified early and lose their adolescence while becoming responsible young adults or they act out their fears and perceived lack of attention by getting into trouble. In one family with two daughters, one became pregnant in high school and the other developed bulimia. Here is how their mother saw it:

> With Barbara getting pregnant, I think part of the reason she got pregnant was because I was, at that point, so tied up in his illness that I really put her on a back burner for a lot

of months. And she began to react by skipping school a lot and finally becoming pregnant. I'm not sure she didn't get pregnant on purpose. I think it was her way of reacting to the way I was reacting to the MS. She was not with a good group of kids and she was doing a lot of running around, and it was just easier for me to say, "Go!" And when the school called to complain about her missing all those classes, at that point I realized this kid is crying for attention. And I made an effort to pay attention to what she was doing and I think it was too late. I think she was already pregnant.

My middle daughter told us this fall that she is bulimic, which nobody noticed, and that took a while for me to accept. Although, again, I knew it, there were signs, but I couldn't deal with it. We got her into counseling and medication. The whole thing is I don't think the MS caused it, but the tension in the house.

In a family with disability, there is relatively little energy left to deal with children's problems. Sometimes the children feel that they can't ask very much of their parents as they see how emotionally and physically stressed the parents are. Barbara's not going to school was not noticed because her parents were distracted by the disease; they had no energy to cope with her problems. One is apt to see children of disabled parents in more difficulties than children from a normal home, both as a reaction to the added family stress and to the lack of parental energy.

On the other hand, children also grow and flourish under the adversity of parental disability. There is a great deal of strength and resilience in this family. Despite their father's illness and increasing disability, their daughter's illegitimate child, and the bulimia, this is still a very close, warm, and supportive family. The well-springs of strength stem in part from their strong religious views and the strength and determination of the mother to keep the family intact. Children can survive and grow under adverse conditions;

what they cannot sustain is indifference, and as long as they feel cared for, they will respond and grow, and what is readily apparent with this family is that as a problem was identified they took immediate action. The children responded well. The bulimia is gone and that daughter is a working professional very close to her family; Barbara lives nearby and the grandchild is a delight.

What parents have to deal with is their own guilt that they are not devoting enough energy and time to the parenting to sustain their children. They also often worry themselves sick that the child might also get ill. Probably the most devastated able-bodied spouse I ever met was the mother of a 25-year-old daughter shortly after her child had been diagnosed as having MS. There is no pain to match that.

Here is John's view of the effects of his wife's Lupus on his two young daughters:

> The biggest effect in our family has been emotionally. We all tend to erupt a little more than we would normally so that the pressures on everybody are greater. It's all verbal screaming, so maybe it's a good thing you get it out of your system and go on to the next thing, whereas, if you didn't do it that way, God only knows how you would get those frustrations out. But it makes for a rocky time.
>
> They can't always understand why we are not like every other family. Fortunately, the physical aspects of the disease, since the surgery, has only had a momentary effect on our lives. The most difficult thing with the disease has been the emotional and psychological aspect of it.
>
> While she was in the hospital, of course, it was extremely tough trying to take care of the two kids, who at that time, were about nine and five, because I was spending so much of the time at the hospital; because she was in such bad shape. I don't know the effect of all of this on my kids. I am a little concerned about the effect on them; the little one who was in first grade that year—we knew it was a severe effect on her

at that time because she had, thank God, an excellent teacher in school who gave her the tender loving care that her mother couldn't give her because she was either too sick or in the hospital. I suspect that when my wife was in the hospital, I gave my older daughter more responsibility than I should have, and possibly turned to the younger one because I was more concerned about how she would handle it and felt the older one would understand. And I wonder now if that is not manifesting itself because my older one will blow up over the silliest damn thing and yell that, "You don't like me, you like my younger sister so much better." I'm getting the feeling that there is a sibling rivalry here that is growing much more than it should. I can't base it on what is happening today, so I go back in my mind: does it go back to when her mom was in the hospital, and because I screwed up and did not give her as much attention and loving—that she could it handle it better than her younger sister? That is one of the things you have to deal with. Here is the guilt. When this thing was really active, there was extreme pressure and you have to start second guessing yourself by saying, "Should I have done something different?" You finally have to say to yourself, "Look, you did it the best you can do it. There was nobody there that laid out the plan for you."

The other thing you worry about; is there a hereditary factor? Not a lot is known about it, so having two daughters we are extremely concerned about that. No question that shortly after she was diagnosed that was the paramount question in our minds; "What have we wrought on our daughters?"

In John's narrative, we can see again how everyone in a family is affected by one person being ill. Everyone has to fill the gap made by the ill person, although the brunt of it will generally be borne by the well spouse. The effects on the children are less clearly defined. It is hard to know how the illness in a parent affects young children who cannot articulate their feelings. There certainly seems to be a great deal of anger floating around in John's family; anger is endemic to chronic illness. It is not so much a matter that it is present in families as it is a matter of how it is handled. In this family, they shout at one another and "blow off steam." Healthy families will acknowledge the anger and support the right of everyone to feel and experience their own rage. Less healthy families repress the anger, which often leads to displacement and to depression. Everyone in a family that contains a person who is chronically ill has a right to be angry. They are cheated of so many things. They feel the enormous pressure of the disease which is distorting their ability to lead a normal life. To blow off steam is not unhealthy, as John noted. The family needs to recognize the source of the anger and then, at some point, direct the anger into productive channels. It is not clear yet what the children are doing with their anger. Counseling can often be effective in these situations by giving the family permission to be angry, then developing acceptable means of expressing the anger, and ultimately channeling it into useful behavior. It requires a sensitive and caring counselor. The people, both shadow people and "patients" that I have met and written about, never need pity (It always makes me angry whenever I think anyone is pitying me or my wife.). What they do need is to be listened to, valued, and to feel that people and society in general care about them. It is a measure of our maturity, both as individuals and as a society, to be caring and compassionate to the chronically ill.

In addition to assuming adult responsibilities early, there is also the problem of identification. A teenage child's notions of how an adult functions stems from his or her in-family experience with the same sex parent. The parent becomes a model for the teenager. How does a teenage boy, for example, model himself after a father who is tired all the time and who can no longer work or drive? Or what model of female adulthood does a young girl have formed from a mother in a wheelchair able to do very little?

Here is one adult daughter's descripton of her mother's MS:

My Mother is the only female role model I've had and now I see her dying by inches. I worry constantly about me getting MS. There are nights when I have to wake up my husband to give me a hug: I'm so scared. Recently I had a tingling sensation in both my arms and I was sure it was MS. Actually it was just stress.

The fear of getting the parental illness plagues the dreams of many a child of disability. A mistake parents often make is to withhold information from their children in order to save them from the pain and worry of the disease process. Children are always aware of the anxiety level in the home and if they are forced to rely on their own fantasies, they are apt to construct scenarios much more grim than the reality. One wonders what guilty thoughts, based on poorly understood facts plague children's dreams. Children need to be "validated" by being included in the family process of coming to grips with the challenge posed by the disease. One child I interviewed was very angry that she was not told about her father's MS and, therefore, was not understanding his "strange" behavior. At times she thought he was drinking too much and at other times she thought he was "going crazy." Her ignorance caused her a lot of guilt when she was finally told about the disease, and anger at her parents for not telling her sooner.

It is not uncommon to find in children of disability resentment or a feeling of being cheated. The daughter, for example, not being able to dance with her father at the college social feels both cheated and grief-stricken for the loss of her father as she knew him. There are so many things that her friends are able to do easily with their parents that are now denied to her. There is so much, that most children can take for granted that she no longer can.

Children of disability also have to handle their friends' reaction to their parents. One time when Cari and I visited my son at college, he agonized over whether he should explain his mother's obvious difficulties in walking to his fraternity brothers before they met her, or wait until afterwards and allow them to ask questions. It was an acute dilemma for him; I'm thankful that he didn't request us to come late at night to be smuggled into his room unnoticed. To a certain extent, all parents are an embarrassment to an adolescent, but the child with a disabled parent suffers acutely. Their parents are really different in ways that are not considered socially desirable.

There is a plus side to this as well. My children have felt that since the diagnosis of MS in our family, there has been more openness, that the family has been closer and they have been allowed more independence earlier. They resent, at times, the increased responsibilities they have had to bear, but they also feel more compassion. I delight in watching my boys with my wife. They are very solicitous in offering her assistance when she needs it. We have all had to assume household responsibilities, learning how to vacuum the house and do the wash quite early. I think Cari and I always encouraged our children to participate fully in the running of the house (I remember when she was getting her Masters' degree, each child was required to prepare one meal a week). The MS pushed up the assumed chores a bit and all of our children left home capable of managing a household. Having a parent with a disability also helps a child get his or her priorities in order. Somehow life's pettiness drops out. Although there is still anger floating around in our family, it seems less tied to the little things of living. We are all able to be more direct and honest about our feelings than we were before the illness. In large part, I think this is a function of my wife and coming to grips with our own issues around her disease and always trying to be open with our children about it.

I think there is also a greater appreciation of me. My children have been much more supportive and concerned about me. When I go on trips, they take on some of my chores and check that things are going well. They also recognize that they are next in line for assuming responsibility for their disabled mother if I can no longer do it. My children are a wonderful source of support for me, but I also know that I must not rely on them. They have their own busy lives to lead, and I must not let them become prisoners of the disability. Children can never own the problems in quite the same way the spouse does, nor should they. The child's biological task is to leave the home and start their own family. To remain to take care of an ailing parent can rob them of their birthright.

We do know that children are sensitive barometers of family stress. All writers on the subject agree that life is stressful for the child of a disabled parent, but the stress can work either way. It can be a maturing factor and produce a responsible child or it can lead to neglect and become a springboard for delinquent behavior. It seems to me that children's success or lack of it is almost always a function of how well the parents are coping with the disease process. When the parents are able to get the disease in perspective so it is no longer dominating their every waking thought and consuming their psychic and physical energy, then they can devote time to their children. Until this happens, the children (especially in the early stages of diagnosis) are pretty much on their own. If there was strength in the family to begin with, then the children can survive and even flourish. In weaker family systems, the children and family itself may not be able to survive without considerable scarring. The effect of parental chronic illness on the adult child is also variable depending in large part on that child's designated role in the family and how close both physically and emotionally that child is to the parent.

Joanne, age 55, is a married mother of two children and a working professional whose widowed mother died of Alzheimer's disease 10 years ago.

> My mother was living alone in her home in Connecticut. My father had died ten years before. I was living in New Jersey at the time and my sister, my only sibling, was living in Long Island. We became aware of the problem very rapidly, which I think means that she had covered it up for many years. She was 79 at the time and the first recollection I have of it was shock, absolute shock. We had a house in Vermont and we always took her up there for Thanksgiving and Christmas. Actually the fall before that, my daughter had gone down to visit her and reported some strange behavior. She said my mother was slicing cabbage and putting it in the toaster. But my mother seemed to be doing fine the rest of the time, and our visits during the year were very short, only an hour or two and just phone calls. So we didn't think anything was wrong. Thanksgiving was awful. I picked her up to go to Vermont. The whole way up she kept saying, "Have I ever been there before?" And she had been up there for years. Just completely disoriented. She knew who I was and who the kids were, but she didn't know where the house was. I remember calling my sister and telling her it was not good. In January, a neighbor of my mother called and said my

mother couldn't handle it anymore; retrospectively we saw her checkbook was a mess and the house was falling apart. So we decided to move her. In February, we got her an apartment near my sister. The moving was hard; probably the hardest part of the whole thing is that you had to con her into doing things.

We had to take the car away from her because she shouldn't drive anymore so we had to lie by telling her that you couldn't get a license in New York after you are eighty. Then we had to take over the money because she couldn't manage that anymore. Then she began to wander. My nephew found her lost one day in the middle of the road, she was about five blocks from her house. Another time she was found in a median strip of a major highway. Some days she would put on three or four dresses and, as I recall, I think there were hallucinations. And at this time she wasn't clear who I was. She kept confusing me with an old friend of hers. Anyway that lasted about five months. This was a very rapid decline and in some way it was very fortunate.

Anyway, it was just getting dangerous. My mother was eating most of her meals at my sister's, which was also disruptive for my sister; she had several children. So then we came to the hardest part of it all, trying to find a nursing home for her. None of the homes wanted her. Finally we did find a place and talked my mother into it but when we got there she decided she didn't like it. I don't know if she knew who I was but she yelled at my sister that she would not stay here. They wouldn't keep her for more than a week. She was wandering in rooms and she just wouldn't stay. It was such a hard time. There was just no place for her and she was so physically healthy. I think one thing they did to control her was to drug her.

Anyway, we finally had to put her into a state hospital which was the only place that would take her. Our big fear was the psychiatric evaluation she needed to get placed into the elderly, senile ward, which wasn't bad. But in order to get through the process, she had to stay in a general ward unit; we were afraid she would be abused by other patients. That was our big fear. She was at the state hospital about eight months and went downhill very fast. The whole process took about three years from when we became aware of her illness to when she died. You always wonder if her husband had been alive, would she have maintained her faculties longer?

Her mother had the very same thing at the very same age, which leaves me and my sister not feeling too good. Should we live and be healthy to that age, we may have the same problem, which scares the hell out of me. Then I keep saying, "If I'm lucky to live that long."

There was so much of a feeling of sadness and loss, and the way I cope with things is to get very busy. A lot of your energy gets used up in trying to do things so you don't have to think about it. I don't think there was any guilt. If there was, it was probably that my sister took more of the burden than I did, but then I took more when my father was sick. So I did feel bad for her. I don't think my mother would have expected anything different than what we had done. There just weren't many options. Given our lifestyle, there was no way she could have moved in with us and if she had, I don't think she could have stayed long. I guess one of the reasons you don't feel guilt in placing someone in a nursing home in the very last stages is that they seem to be so unaware of what is happening that they are not going to sense the loss you would as with a physically handicapped person. My father was in a nursing home for a while, and that was okay in our family. The real sadness is that you couldn't really talk to her about it. That probably bothers me more than anything. I'm convinced that at some point in time, she really knew what was happening to her. The crazy thing too is that someone has really died two years ago, in essence, yet their actual death is still a horrible process. I don't know what you hang on to. You hang on to something. The difficulty is then of getting that memory of the last stages out of your mind. The impressions are so strong. That's not what you want to remember about them. It's hard to bring them back the way they were. It takes a long time when you remember them, not to remember them the way they were at the end. It happens eventually. It takes time.

Joanne demonstrates a lot of the coping problems of the adult child of disability. One is the physical distance from the parent that has to be negotiated. In some ways distance is a blessing because it lets you "forget" about the loss while you go about your life and are not exposed to the disabled parent on a daily basis. On the other hand, you have to deal with the guilt of not doing your share. Joanne can assuage her guilt by recalling that she had been more actively involved in her father's care than her sister. There is also the shock that happens to the physically distant child each time he or she encounters the disabled parent; the decline is so much more obvious to the child that each visit requires a whole new adjustment process.

The other difficulty that all children of disability have, but which I think is especially true of Alzheimer's children, is the grim specter of the genetic component of the disease which haunts their peace of mind. In this case both Joanne's mother and grandmother had become ill at age 79, which is terrifying to both Joanne and her sister. There is nothing that anyone can say that would take away the fear; it is something they live with constantly.

In Joanne's case, the normal adult role reversal had pretty much taken place by the time her mother became ill, although it was still shocking for her to see her mother as a dependent child. It is easier for adult children who have been on their own to make the caretaker transition than for children who are still dependent or still living at home. For most families the decision to institutionalize the patient is very painful.

For many families, the decision to institutionalize is an economic one. At $4,000+ a month, most families cannot afford to keep a family member in a nursing home for long, so they attempt to do it themselves, usually at horrendous cost to the health and welfare of the rest of the family. The laws are such that families must reduce themselves to a poverty status before they can begin to "afford" a nursing home so when faced with the twin prospects of poverty or exhaustion, most families opt for exhaustion; the literature is replete with instances where the able-bodied spouse, especially of the dementing illness, needed psychiatric care and hospitalization. Depression and exhaustion are the two most common components of the caretakers.

Joanne and her sister were able to institutionalize their mother relatively easily because of their prior positive experience of their father's nursing home. Institutionalization fits within the culture of this particular family; the decision to institutionalize is very complex involving a host of variables. Among them are the amount of family strain, family finances, the support structure of the family and the health of the primary caretaker.[10] Dementia in particular is an illness striking the patient at the core of his or her humanness, altering the hallmarks of personality and intelligence. The worm of the disease burrows deeply within and destroys a person's substance leaving only the empty husk of the person for others to view. The body remains the same, at least in the early stages, but the mind and personhood are gone as family members remember it. There is psychological death long before physical death. There are no rituals to help the family through the mourning. It is a never ending struggle for family members of dementia patients to try to keep fresh the memory of what used to be while dealing with the present reality which bears no resemblance, in the ways that matter, to the person they knew.

Nuland[3] (opcit) caught the problem so well when

he wrote:

> It often seems as though the families of Alzheimer's patients
> are sidetracked from the broad sunlit avenues of ongoing
> life, remaining trapped for years each in its own excruciat-
> ing cul-de-sac, the only rescue comes with the death of a per-
> son they love. And even then, the memories and the dreadful
> toll drag on and from these the release can only be partial. A
> life that has been lived and a shared sense of happiness and
> accomplishments are ever after seen through the smudged
> glass of its last few years. For the survivors, the concourse of
> existence has forever become less bright and less direct (pp.
> 105).

Joanne was remembering the pain of an Alzheimer parent. John is living it. John, age 54, is a
physician who is married to a nurse and is the father
of two children. He is the fourth of six children. His
mother, who was divorced 30 years ago, has lived for
the past 17 years in the house adjoining John's proper-
ty. This house was bought by John specifically for his
mother. His siblings live in the surrounding community. Two years ago his mother, age 78, was diagnosed
as having Alzheimer's disease.

> I guess my mother has had the disease for the past five
> years but we had it diagnosed about two years ago. I guess
> we just didn't want to know about it; things were wrong for
> a long time. She used to deposit her social security checks
> and then she began to cash them and the money kept disap-
> pearing. The people at the market told my sister that she
> was giving them $100 bills to pay for her food.
> We have taken turns taking care of her. It is very hard
> and emotionally exhausting. In the morning I get up and
> make her coffee and see that she takes her pills. We have
> turned off her stove. When she asks about the stove, we tell
> her it's broken and we'll get it fixed. I go to work and she
> calls my sister, who is my office manager, and wants to
> know what she is supposed to do that day. My sister tells
> her what her day is going to be like, which on Monday,
> Wednesday, and Friday is to go to day care. On Tuesdays

and Thursdays each of my brothers takes a day and comes over to the house and takes her to their homes or out for dinner. My other sister comes over and helps her get dressed. I wouldn't do that although the other day she answered the door in her underwear—this in a very vain Italian woman.

She is very paranoid about money and about food. She always wants to know when she is going to eat. Yesterday she came out to the yard where I was working and this would be a typical conversation: "I want to go shopping only I don't have any money." "Mom, you don't need money. Ruth will take you shopping and give you money." Ten minutes later she says the same thing over and over again and it just drives you crazy. It is a catch 22. If you give her money, she just loses it and then accuses you of taking it. It is exhausting being around her.

One of the things with my mother is that I have always cared for her. She never had a lot of joy in her life; she never had a good relationship with my father and I always wanted to make her happy and I used to try to make her happy. When she developed Alzheimer's disease, for the first time in my life I realized that not only could I not make her happy now, but a lot of the things I tried to make her happy with previously couldn't have made her happy. My mother, for example, always complained about not having enough money. If she had enough money she could travel. I used to believe her so I gave her money but she still never travelled. What Alzheimer's has done is taught me a lot about life and personalities in general. It's taught me that money is not as important as your physical, and more important, your mental outlook on life.

In some ways it has also brought our family closer. My brothers and sisters all love her but in a different way. Originally my youngest brother and youngest sister wanted to put her in a nursing home. My mother has been seeing a psychiatrist and she (the psychiatrist) has been preparing us for putting her in a nursing home. None of us wants this because they drug them there. When my youngest brother first found out she had Alzheimer's, he got very sympathetic and went to see her two and three times a week taking her out for supper. Then he got drained by the whole thing. He did a complete reversal, saying that he couldn't handle it anymore than once a week, but he felt she should be in a nursing home. Now he's going back to the point where he feels he couldn't put her in a nursing home. My expectations are that my mother will probably live another 10 years and that some day she will be in a nursing home and that our personalities and mental toughness are going to be tried over and over again.

What keeps me going is getting away from it and sharing the load. I could never do it by myself. In spite of what little others may have done it's more than they've done the rest of her life. My oldest brother has been taking at least one session a week. Before that he would come only once in a while and might watch the golf match on TV at her house, and when the golf match was over, he would leave—just sort of like fulfilling his obligation. So he's doing more than he ever did. I honestly don't know how I would do it if my wife wasn't good—although just to give you an idea of everyone's threshold: My mother was downstairs with my wife at lunch and she started in with my wife wanting to know where she would get some money. So my wife tried to carry on a rational conversation with her, which you do because she looks rational and you think you can get across to her. (You know this has been almost two years and there are still some days you think she is perfectly normal.) Then there's a fight and the next thing I knew my mother slammed the door. When I came in, my wife was very angry and very upset. So I called up my mother and she said, "I can't remember what I said to your wife. I know it was something and I got her angry." Then she said, "I don't have anything in the house to eat tonight." I said, "You're going to eat here." She said, "I can't come back because I was mean to your wife." And this goes on all the time. Some days my wife can take it and some days she can't. The same for me—when you can't take it, you have to back off. I see this in my sister at work. She doesn't even know when she's doing it. I don't know when I'm doing it. Generally I think my sister Ruth, myself, and my wife would probably get the brunt of it. With six of us, it's still a problem. I had a patient whose husband had Alzheimer's disease and she tried to take care of him at home and she wound up in a mental hospital.

> We got help for my mother. We got a woman to come in
> and watch her. My mother made it so miserable for her that
> she had to leave. When you talk to people they all have a
> solution but they haven't dealt with it. I would do the same
> thing. There is no solution—absolutely no solution. It's one
> thing to see something from the outside but you don't know
> what it is until you live it. I think I've become a much more
> compassionate physician now.

Listening to John describe life with his mother,
one is struck again by what an enormous strain it is
to live with a dementing relative. Although he says
you can't really know it unless you live with it, one
can get a sense of the total internal and physical
drain that his mother's illness causes in the whole
family. There is no way only one person can manage
to cope with this disorder and John feels fortunate
that it is spread somewhat among the six children. It
never works out evenly in any family and this family
is no exception. John and his sister Ruth bear the
brunt of the care, with the others supplementing
where possible. The tensions and anger in the family
are enormous. It is so easy for the anger about the
situation of a dementing parent to get displaced on a
sibling who is not "doing his share." It is so hard to
know what is a proper "share." This family has, for
the time being, achieved a precarious balance by
Ruth and John filling in the slack caused by a failure
of a sibling to fulfill his or her obligation. By some
strange family alchemy, John has always been his
mother's designated savior. Each child is born into a
different family and each establishes his or her own
role. Alzheimer's disease has not changed John's role;
if anything it has intensified and expanded it. Families do not become different entities when stressed by
chronic illness; they tend to become more solidified in

their structure. The tendencies that were always within the family become exaggerated and members usually fulfill their role expectation that were developed early in the family history. John will probably always feel like the child who is most responsible for his mother's welfare, although he has learned, as a result of the disease, that he never could make her happy.

Jan, age 31, is a professional woman who was a student of mine. She is the only daughter of five children. Her mother has MS and her father is a long standing alcoholic. Early on in the family she was parentified to conspire with her mother in enabling the father to be an alcoholic. Her brothers were passive and she was the child who cleaned up the mess and made excuses for him. When her mother was diagnosed with MS ten years ago, her father "fell apart." Everyone looked to Jan to fulfill her expected role in the family. She tried to do this, while going to school and having also recently gotten married. Finally she recognized that she could no longer do it all and she has been actively trying to set boundaries with her family members. It is hard for her to know what is the appropriate amount for her to do and when to say "no." Whenever she does set a boundary it is always tinged with guilt because she is not fulfilling her designated family role—it engenders anger in the other family members because she is violating their expectations. But since she has been setting her limits her brothers are becoming more active as the family system accommodates to her reduced savior role. Jan has needed a lot of help in setting these boundaries and counseling has been effective for her.

For adult children of disability, a parent's illness is a mixed bag. There is a great deal of loss and pain that nothing can take away; what children try to retain is the memory of their parents as vital, competent persons, something very difficult to accomplish, especially in the terminal stages of the disease when their parents are so ravaged. Perhaps the ultimate act of childhood is the burying of your parents; for the children of disability, it is not always clear when death takes place. What is clear is that they are called upon to become compassionate, caring adults at an early age; and this is something which many of these children seem to accomplish very well.

CHAPTER 4

Parents of Disability

In the normal course of events, children begin life as totally dependent beings and if the parents do their task properly, they create independent adults who no longer need them. That is the biological mandate of parenthood. There should come a point in which parents expect their children to become more vibrant and more capable than they. In many low income families children are seen as a precious commodity providing free labor and a social security system for eventually taking care of the aging parents. The developmental task of midlife adults is adjusting to the aging of their parents and eventually becoming caregivers to them. This usually occurs at the time that adults cease actively parenting their own children and then turn around and parent their parents; this is the so-called "sandwich generation."

It is probably every parent's worst nightmare to think of having to bury a child. In actuality, up to the beginning of this century, the death of a child was fairly commonplace; one has only to wander through an 18th or 19th century graveyard to see the large number of gravestones devoted to children, to recognize how precarious childhood was prior to the development of modern medical technology. Parents had large families in the expectation that only a few children would survive to adulthood. Medical technology has changed all of that. Now, in the United States, families are smaller and there is a strong and reasonable expectation that children will survive and outlive their parents.

For a parent to become increasingly more competent than his adult child is a violation of the way things are supposed to be. It causes anger and a great deal of pain. Parents of chronically ill children, day in and day out, have to confront the twin horrors of decreasing competency in their child, and since many of these chronic illnesses shorten the life span, there is a very real possibility of out-living their child. They also experience a terrible feeling of helplessness—parents are supposed to make things better for a hurting child, and these parents can't. The father of a son with severe multiple sclerosis:

> It feels to me that now I am raising my child for a second time. I did it once successfully and my wife and I were really enjoying being free of child rearing responsibilities and now he has moved back home getting progressively less able and we are at a loss as to what to do.

Parents, unlike spouses, have no choice in the matter; we don't choose our children, nor can we ever divorce them. Some parents physically and psychologically can distance themselves from the problem, but at some level all parents must psychologically own the chronic illness in their child if for no other reason than the guilt they feel for having in some way caused the illness—either through the transmission of a defective gene or through a failure to fulfill their parental responsibility of safeguarding the health of the child. Because of their underlying guilt, parents tend to "own" the disease in ways that a spouse or a child of disability do not. Parents, especially the older parents who are not living in the home with the chronically ill child, get stuck in denial. They are filled with fear, guilt, and grief to such a strong measure that the only way they can cope is by denying the disease.

In the early stages of the disease my mother-in-law, despite every explanation, was still hoping that there was a possible cure for MS and could not understand why we didn't pursue more medical or pseudo-medical cures. When her daughter had periods in which her walking was a bit more stable, then she thought the improvement was permanent and she despaired when Cari had to use a wheelchair. My wife, on the other hand, would try to hide the ravages of the disease process from her mother so as not to further upset her but she cannot do it anymore and they are both being forced to take a more realistic view of the disease now that it has progressed beyond the early stages and the effects of the MS are so apparent to everyone.

My mother-in-law has often said that she would gladly trade legs with her daughter and I am sure many parents of disabled children feel the same way. Parents who discover that their child who is living at home, has a chronic illness, have a dual problem of coping with the guilt, fear, and anger that all parents of chronically ill children experience, but also helping to manage the disease process in their child while, at the same time, negotiating the formidable issues of raising an adolescent child to adulthood. Let us look at one such family.

The Family

James, age 55, is the director of a community service organization; his wife, Nancy, age 56, is a recently retired teacher. They have three children. Karen, age 30, is a nurse; Michael, age 29, is recovering from a serious auto injury; and Emily, age 28, is also a nurse. Both Karen and Emily have juvenile diabetes.

The Mother's Story

They both were diagnosed when they turned twelve. With Karen, we never expected anything serious. I just thought she was having problems becoming a teenager. Looking back on it, it seems so apparent that she was ill; she was losing weight, always thirsty, and always going to the bathroom, but we also couldn't communicate. She was just withdrawn; it just seemed as though she was tuning us out. She looked bad, but we thought it was because she was doing crazy things—her hair was long and she didn't wash it—we were concerned with behavioral things. We were considering counseling. It wasn't until the teacher called me from school and thought I should get a physical for her, and that really upset me. I couldn't get an appointment for three weeks, and I had to insist because we couldn't go anywhere with her. They finally gave me an appointment, and I don't know what made me say, "I want her checked for diabetes." My father and maternal uncle had diabetes, but my father's didn't develop until he was 65—but I did bring in urine samples from everyone—but never thought she might have diabetes. I remember I had the last appointment of the day and they sent the specimen to the lab at the hospital. I called James and said, "I think you'd better come over. I think there is trouble." It turned out her blood sugar level was 55—near the coma level.

They didn't know how she was functioning. They didn't let her go home or anything; they just put her in the hospital. I was very alarmed. I remember telling Karen, "Well, at least you can live with this—other things you can't." Her roommate at the hospital was diagnosed as having leukemia.

It was hard, because at the time Karen was diagnosed (eighteen years ago) they were very regimented and came down very hard on children. They told them they could never have candy and could never have sweets. Karen has since told us the story that the first time she had a piece of candy, she really did not know but that she might die and she still ate it and then when nothing happened, she ate another piece. Her eating habits are still poor. There again is her old habit of always testing the limits. She tested all the time. I finally had to realize that diabetes is her problem, and you can't protect them that much.

A year later we found that Emily had diabetes, too, but she didn't have any symptoms at all. We were checking everybody, and her urine sample showed up positively. When we put her in the hospital, they gave her insulin, and that stimulated her pancreas. They told us that she would eventually have to have insulin injections. They didn't know how long this would last. She went for another year and they (the doctors) decided that she needed the injections. They were very calm about it, and Karen gave Emily the injections and taught her how to do it. In fact, I never gave the girls an injection; they always handled it themselves.

Karen follows her own plan and seems to do just fine. She's never had any more problems—at least any that I know of. Emily, evidently, is the more brittle of the two of them; she tries very hard to eat correctly and be in control, and she's had practically everything that comes along. One time passing out in the morning from too little sugar before she was going to school, I just found her in a heap. She's had diabetes retinopathy; she's had laser surgery already; she had that four years ago—before that she went to a kidney specialist; she's also had some sensation difficulty. Each one of these complaints is scary, because once you begin to know something about diabetes, you begin to realize that it is not the diabetes itself or the management of it; it's the consequence of uncontrolled diabetes that leads to stroke or to blindness and to loss of lives through circulation problems and kidney failure that are life threatening or severely debilitating. So those complications begin to be the anxiety points about the disease. I still worry about Karen; even though she hasn't had any symptoms, she can always get them. Even if you maintain tight control, you can still get serious complications. It's always been a puzzle to me why Karen had done so well and Emily seems to get everything. It's painful when those things happen, yet you feel you can't really acknowledge that those things are painful. You have to sort of be supportive of them. I think I do all right with the brittle symptom, but the kids think I overreact.

All of this has affected our marriage, because we became so over-focused on the kids. James took over all the responsibility and I let him, even though I knew that wasn't the best thing, but I didn't have a better answer—it just was a very difficult time. I can remember Michael asking all the time if he was going to get diabetes, and I couldn't promise him he wouldn't. I hadn't expected Emily to be diabetic.

What I am glad about is that I don't think either girl limited herself because of the diabetes. I know Karen was upset at one point because she couldn't get into the armed services—I don't know if she even really wanted to be there or just wanted to test the limits. I know that Emily pushed herself harder to do things because of the diabetes. She always insisted on doing things. There was a church group that had an overnight bike trip. I thought they were crazy to let her go because of her diabetes. I really admired her; she was the last one, but she did it. I didn't want to let her go, but she was determined to go. After Karen, we learned that we couldn't control them.

I think the diabetes strengthened our marriage. I think, when you get a lot of stress, either it makes you stronger or you don't make it. For me, I think you only have one go-around in this life, and you need to make the most of it. I think the diabetes, as awful a disease as it is, has strengthened all of us.

Father's Story

All the symptoms we tuned into were the behavioral ones, and I felt badly when we found out she had a physical problem all along. There was a personality change in a short period of time. We didn't have good information about diabetes—the doctors were telling us to get control of this at a time when our kids were adolescents. My general attitude always was, "OK. If you have a problem, you have to confront it, and you have to know what to do about it and to manage it as best you can." What I really got into was, "OK, here is what we are going to do. First of all, you are going to do all the right things all the time." Instead of coming off as caring and wanting to help, I came off as more dictatorial and parental. This was to an adolescent who was basically wanting to change that role anyway and who herself was trying to integrate the notion of having a lifelong and life-threatening disease that she didn't understand well either. So she and I got into some very severe rebellion, resistance, anger, hostility kind of stuff. The focal point of her illness was the confrontation between us—the contention over who was in charge of her. It did exacerbate the adolescent issue. For us, the adolescent issues became life and death issues, at least as how we perceived them. I have been so afraid of the complications of diabetes.

In the beginning, I thought it was just a matter of main-taining tight control; I used to think that if you were remiss on any occasion, you would have complications, and there is the tendency to feel that this is the punishment for having failed to maintain it perfectly. I know now that that is not true. That was the parental rigidity I was on—I had to make sure they do it perfectly. That is what I thought I could do for them, and, of course, I couldn't, if there was ever any such possibility. That's why I got into such conflict with Karen. It was a terribly painful time for her in terms of all of the things she was trying to cope with. When we recently asked her about that time, she told us she was thinking of running away, but when she thought about running away, she knew she couldn't because of the diabetes—because she knew she could get in real trouble!

Emily was more compliant and easier, but I think I made all my big mistakes in such a grand manner with Karen—she led the way. I eased off with Emily. It just got so very bad with Karen. It was clear we weren't communicat-ing at all, and she wasn't communicating with the doctor either. The doctor was giving her lectures and she wasn't lis-tening, and she wasn't complying at all with what the doctor wanted, and I was getting frantic. And finally, she said she didn't like to go to that doctor because it was not her doctor, it was my doctor: "She talks to you rather than me." So she wanted another doctor, and she didn't want me to be in-volved in it. We found a doctor who was involved in diabetes who was a diabetic himself. When I contacted him and told him the situation, he said he would see Karen, but that she personally would need to call to make the appointment and that Karen would need to talk to him directly. So I came home and told her what the offer was and she called and they talked on the phone. He told her that he would see her and they could decide together whether he would continue to see her. He did insist that I come on the first visit and Karen agreed reluctantly. And so we went in and he saw her alone for a good long while; after which he came out and said to me (this was while Karen was sitting in the corner with her arms crossed, looking like her resolutely unhappy self), "Well, Karen and I had a good visit, and I think I understand her medical condition. There appear to be two people with a problem here. Karen's diabetes is a medical problem and she can manage that problem. I will take responsibility for managing her diabetes, and you are relieved of any responsibility except for getting her here and paying the bills. If you have any questions about diabetes or about her care, you are free to call me."

He granted me absolution—right off the bat he said to me, "I know lots about diabetes, but I can't manage it for her. So all I can do is give her the basic information, which she has a good grasp of—and then it's her problem. If I can't take care of it for her, you certainly can't." That's exactly what I needed to hear in terms of information and attitude, and that did a great deal to ease the tension for me and in our whole family—at that point in time we were nearly all basket cases. Because, you know, in addition, we had three very-close-in-age adolescent children, and we were two working, professional parents. It was a very scary time.

Looking back on it, I don't know how we survived it. I think the answer lies in our attitude—which for me is, if life hands you lemons, then make lemonade out of it—and the fact that we had each other. I always knew that Nancy would listen to me—she could always hear me and, at times, I think she was the only one.

Since the adolescent period we've had some awfully, awfully difficult times. Emily's problems sometimes came on her so quickly and unexpectedly. Probably the worst single time was a call we got in the morning from Emily. She had just moved into an apartment and we hadn't been there yet and didn't know exactly where it was. We didn't have an address or a phone number, and she had moved the day before. We had gotten this phone call, and it was an almost unintelligible voice on the phone, and then I realized it was Emily—she was incoherent and in-and-out. She made it known to me that she was on the floor and she just crawled to get the phone and she had no feeling in her arm, and she was obviously struggling to be coherent but not really—and I realized, here is my kid on the other end of the phone in desperate need of attention, and I didn't know where she was and she couldn't tell me. And I was just on the point of panicking—I was at the point of desperation. I asked her if Karen knew where she was and she told me, yes, because she had helped her move and I realized I didn't even know if Karen was home, but I got Emily to hang up. Fortunately, I got a hold of Karen, and she and her husband drove out and found Emily, and, fortunately, it was just low sugar. If you give her some sugar, she turns right around, but if she doesn't get it, she can die—and that's the awful thing you carry around with diabetes all the time. I guess this is why I am so indulgent with her; whenever she wants to do something, I tell her to just go right ahead—you don't know how much time she has.

Some Thoughts

According to my mother-in-law, to be a mother is to worry; certainly to be the parent of a diabetic child is to worry constantly. The grim, ever-present specter of the diabetic complication continuously haunts the dreams and waking thought of every parent of a diabetic child. In many respects the emotional burden of chronic illness is more difficult for the co-disabled than it is for the person with the illness. The co-disabled, as James had to find out for himself, really have no control over the disease or over the course of the disease; they must wait in the wing frustrated, scared, and sometimes despairing. The person with the illness, while not able to change the course of the disease, is often able to alleviate some of the symptoms by conforming to proper maintenance, that is, by taking insulin and observing the diet. The diabetic at least has the illusion perhaps of being able to control the disease. The parents have absolutely no control; when they try to gain some control, an unhealthy dynamic often occurs around responsibility, as clearly happened in this family.

The issue of control is not confined to parents or to diabetes but occurs in all diseases and with healthy spouses and healthy children as well. No relationship between parent and child is ever simple; chronic illness complicates an already difficult task. Parents with chronically ill children must learn, usually very painfully, that they cannot manage the disease; to attempt to do so will only cause greater pain for them and for their child. Primary responsibility for the management of the disease must be transferred to the child (or spouse, or parent) very early in the course of treatment and then the parent must learn to live with a feeling of impotence. As Nancy noted, "diabetes is her problem" but powerlessness is one of the most difficult feelings to manage; it often leads to an inner rage that has no expression other than deep depression.

For parents there is almost always a great deal of guilt. In my experience, mothers usually feel responsibility for having caused the disease. Mothers traditionally have the role in the family for the health and safety of the children. When a child is ill, the mother often feels that she somehow failed. It is difficult to carry a child for nine months during pregnancy and not have something untoward happen that you can in retrospect blame as the cause of the illness and many mothers have a "guilty secret." They know, even if nobody else does, that they did something to cause the disease. Mothers also seem to take responsibility for all of a child's genes, forgetting that the father contributed his half, too. The burden of guilt for the mother often leads to over-protection ("I let something bad happen once, I am not going to let it happen again.") or to assuming too much responsibility for the treatment of the disease. The mother is also the one parent most inclined to try to fix the child—to make the child whole again.

Maternal guilt then leads to over-commitment to the "I let something bad happen to you, now I'm going to make it up to you" thought. The super-dedicated mother will drop almost everything in her life to try to fix it. Professionals who see this parent in the early stages of diagnosis marvel at how devoted she is and rate her high on any scale of parent effectiveness, however, if you examine a family with a super-dedicated mother several years later, you will often find that the family is in shambles. There are only seven days in a week and twenty four hours in a day and if most of the time is spent with the ill child, then other components of the family system will suffer. In addition to the problems of over-control and consequent tension between parents and child as described by Nancy and James, the families of super-dedicated parents usually have adversely affected siblings and very often marriages that are at risk. Families cannot maintain themselves for long unless there is energy available to do the necessary maintenance tasks to keep the system intact. At times families need time out for fun and they need time to discuss and eventually redefine their roles.

A father's guilt leads to the same unproductive behavior of over-protection and over-management, but the source of the guilt has a different basis than maternal guilt. Fathers usually feel the guilt of being impotent in eliminating the pain that is in the family. A father's role in a traditional family is to stand at the gates and defend his family against any dragons that may be attacking. When family members are ill or hurting, the father sees this as a failure on his part and either he responds with denial and tries to have everyone else in the family deny their feelings of sadness or he tries, as James did, to "solve the problem" and establish control, often with disastrous results.

For parents, the chronically ill child is often perceived as a shared failure and can have a negative impact on the marriage. In the first place so much of the parent's energy is devoted to the child there is little left for the marriage. The child also can be easily triangulated into long simmering areas of marital conflict; it is so easy for the husband, for example, to blame his wife for causing the disease and for her to blame him for not solving the problem. The disease can become a potent weapon in a long established marital war; the disease (or more properly, the reaction to the disease) can become the ultimate weapon leading to the marital Armageddon.

It also works the other way, as in this family where the diabetes ultimately strengthened the marriage; Nancy and James were able to grow, albeit with a great deal of stress and turmoil. Not only is the diabetes a shared failure, it is also a shared challenge that can foster closeness and an appreciation of their mutual strengths and need for each other. I think all the really important things I have learned in life have only come out of stress and turmoil. I wish I could learn the easy way, but my life doesn't seem to be fashioned that way.

Older parents who have produced a viable independent adult also suffers acutely when they have to watch their child slowly deteriorate. One father lamented "you raise your child and think you have done your job and now you have it to do again, only you haven't the energy for it." Mary, a 59-year-old widow, has a 37-year-old daughter who has lupus. Mary's daughter, who was living independently, has recently moved back home because she can no longer work and, therefore, can no longer support herself. Here briefly is her story:

> When Alice told me she had lupus, I didn't know what that meant. I read some things about it and it scared me terribly. I thought I would lose her right away but fortunately it seems to have stabilized. Now she has a visual problem because of the cataracts she got from the treatment and she is just too fatigued to work, she had to move home. This was a terrible blow to her pride and self-esteem. She had a good job and she was independent. Now she is dependent on me— I have to drive her everywhere. Most of her friends have left her. She is depressed most of the time and I worry. Who will take care of her after I'm gone or who will take care of me after I no longer can do for myself. All we have is each other.

Every parent of a disabled child with a chronic, progressive illness is plagued by the question of who will take care of him or her after I am gone. Or as in this case when I am too old to care for myself, much less for my child. Parents who take on the caretaker role again worry about this more than spouses because they are older than a spouse and are closer to being more infirm than a well spouse might be. Often the responsibility for the disabled child falls on the child's sibling. Recently I met with parents of a disabled child who were setting up a trust fund for their child and were seeking a guardian to manage the trust and ultimately their child. At best this is a painful process, at its worst it is an unholy nightmare as parents seek frantically to find someone who can and will take responsibility for their child when they no longer can.

Traditionally family has been the ultimate protector of the disabled and when family can no longer do it then we must have community. In the long run all we have is each other.

CHAPTER 5

Coping

The chronic, progressive diseases described in this book have the following characteristics:

1) They always get worse with an unpredictable course.
2) There is no cure.
3) The cause is unknown, although all seem to have some genetic component and a suspected "trigger" mechanism.
4) They all begin insidiously and are difficult to diagnose.
5) The medical profession offers little but relief of symptoms.
6) Everyone in the family is affected by the disease.

These are all diseases in which the person who has the disease did nothing to merit it. These are diseases that happen to people, to very good people, and there is no one or no thing to blame. In the long run, these diseases teach us how to live with powerlessness or, more importantly, how to retain some control in the face of the inability to change the course of the disease.

I have interviewed many families for this book and I am struck at how universal the stories are. On the surface the families are very different, some just starting out, others with young children at home, and others whose grown children may be out of the house —the specifics may be vastly different but the stories are surprisingly the same.

Underlying families' stories is always the slow acceptance process characterized by denial. Then there is the havoc that ensues in the family as traditional roles become realigned, leading finally, in the more successful families to restructuring of priorities and roles so they can continue to function. The less successful families are always characterized by a lack of communication among the family members. After the initial diagnosis in these families there is a conspiracy of silence characterized by an unwillingness to talk about the disease and an unwillingness to renegotiate family roles. Many of the unsuccessful families that do not end in an overt estrangement, live together in a marital hell characterized by free-floating anger that becomes fixated on minor transgressions and fears and guilts neither articulated nor understood.

There are four distinct phases to the acceptance process although frequently the lines between the phases get blurred as individuals are in the transition process. The stages are: denial, resistance, affirmation, and integration.

Denial is characterized by the concealing of symptoms, the seeking of an authority who will refute the diagnosis, a belief that this is not true, that it couldn't be happening, and an almost fervent holding on to past values and lifestyle. There is a great deal of strength in denial, built in large part on the fear of change or, more specifically, on the insecurity about the ability to cope. Denial, however, can only be maintained for so long because it is constantly assaulted by the evidence of the disease; it also can only be maintained for so long without, in many cases, causing irreparable damage.

The denial mechanism is very sustaining and often is the only thing the identified patient feels that he or she has to keep going. The wife, for example, who watches her husband struggle to put on his clothes, wants to help and facilitate the whole process; it would be so much easier if she did it. To do so would mean an admission that he can't and so her husband consistently refuses help even though it exhausts him to get dressed. This is the "strength" part of the denial even though it is often difficult to live with. (This contrasts with the husband who told his wife, shortly after getting the definitive diagnosis of MS, that "This is my out" as he took to his wheelchair never to walk or work again. Needless to say that marriage did not last long.)

Denial can also be dangerous as in the case of the spouse who continues to drive long past the time it is safe. In this situation, it may be necessary to intervene—it's always a difficult judgement call for the shadow spouse to make. One of the greatest difficulties the spouse has, as with raising a child, is how much control do you give to the patient and how much do you keep. This is especially true in the dementing disorders, but denial can easily cloud the judgement of any person. While it is absolutely essential that you help your spouse maintain his or her independence as long as possible; health and safety considerations must also come into play.

Denial is also very much the lot of the shadow spouse. In the early stages of the disease it is characterized by explaining away the symptoms: later on it is refusing to believe the husband or wife can no longer function adequately. I have met families who did not make necessary adjustments to accommodate the changed realities and a disability rapidly became a handicap. For example, in one family, the wife with MS literally became house bound because nobody would build a ramp so that she could leave the home easily. Everyone in the family was busy maintaining the fiction that she was just as she always had been and nobody seemed to notice that she seldom went out anymore.

In the resistant stage, the individual acknowledges to self but often not to others that there is something wrong but refuses to accept the notion that the disease "will win." This is the pledge (and sometimes the bargain you try to make with "God" at 3:00 A.M.) that you and your spouse are not going to be like "them." You will change your life style; eating healthier, taking vitamins, etc. and you will beat the disease, if not reversing it, then certainly arresting the progression. In this stage of coping, there is an active search for a cure; there is also increased activity in seeking others who have the problem and may have found a treatment for it. There is the often unexpressed belief that somehow you will be a special case and the disease, as manifested in your spouse, will have a much more benign course than predicted by the doctors. Shortly after the diagnosis of MS, Cari ran a 10K race; as much to prove to herself that she could still do it as to state that she was a special case. I can remember her bobbing and weaving to the finish line and my watching her with mixed emotions of pride and embarrassment. My then 9-year-old son was there too and said "I hate to see Mom like this"; all I could do was agree with him. As in denial, this stage is often marked by a refusal to accept help—to do so means you are not "winning."

The third stage is affirmation. At this point there is an acknowledgement that you and your spouse have the disease and the doctors were right. Then you begin the process anew of grieving for the former couple, and for your former life; you are no longer buttressed by denial and resistance. This stage is characterized by a great deal of pain as there is an acceptance of the notion that things will never again be as they were. There is also now a willingness to accept help and publicly acknowledge that there is something wrong. Families begin to educate others about the disease, and often become active in support groups and in public associations that promote information and awareness about the disease. You also begin the lifelong process of rearranging your life's priorities. You acknowledge that your life will never be the same again but it does not have to be a bad one, just different from what you expected.

The fourth and final stage, integration (sometimes referred to as adaptation), is characterized by getting the ramifications of the disease in perspective. It is learning to live with it, and then spending time and energy on other matters. It is integrating the changes caused by the disease into a new life style with changed values. The affirmation and adaptation stages are reached when you realize that "beating" the disease is often a matter of learning to live life to the fullest in the face of the on-going disease process.

The routines of living with a wheelchair-bound person become just that: routines. You are not aware of how much you have adapted your lifestyle to the disability until someone tries to help you out. For me, for example, it became routine to get Cari and her scooter into the adapted van to the point where we don't think about the process until someone tries to do it and we realize then that it is pretty complicated process. We had to learn each step by painful trial and error and now we just do it.

Chronic, progressive illness forces you to confront frightening change on a daily basis, and the acceptance process of moving from denial to resistance to affirmation and ultimately on to adaptation keeps recurring as new challenges emerge. This is at best a sloppy process with no clear demarcation points. Any change (which occurs constantly with these diseases) forces you to go through the cycle again. After much thought and discussion, Cari and I purchased that 3-wheel scooter. I watched the process occur in both of us as we moved through the resistance phase into affirmation. The wheelchair looked, at first, like it was a big "giving up" and meant we had to let go of our resistance to the disease process. It meant admitting to everyone that she was disabled and it would put us in the category of "handicapped couple," which we did not want. I remember not being able to look at the scooters ads that my wife kept leaving on the table. (She was way ahead of me on this one.) And when we finally did get one, it remained in our living room unused for several months. Now we feel we could not survive without it. Recently we purchased a motorized wheelchair to go with our new van and it sits in our living room unused and unloved, and the process begins again.

In actuality, the "scooter" has increased our mobility and Cari's independence, giving us both more life options, but I couldn't force us to move any faster than we were psychologically ready to go. When we are ready for the wheelchair, we'll do what we have to do, and I have to curb my impatience at wanting to get the job done. Timing is all; the use of the scooter came as a relief rather than a defeat, although it is still, at times painful for me to see her in it because it is also the MS objectified.

Individuals will vary as to the degree and speed by which they can get to the adaptation stage. Some families never get there; they seem forever stuck in the denial and resistance stages which seems to them to be the only possible coping strategy; they are paralyzed in their fear. Others move through the process very rapidly, seeming to skip stages. I think the key to successful adaptation lies in the self-confidence of families. When an individual feels secure in his or her ability to cope, it becomes easier to assume the psychological risk of giving up the pseudo comfort of denial and assuming the responsibilities demanded by the affirmation and adaptation stages of the coping process. The acceptance stages are not firmly fixed points as in climbing a mountain, once gained never lost, but rather a very fluid series of points in time in which even very successfully adapted couples move into earlier stages. I, for example, still find it very hard to attend a meeting where I know there will be people with multiple sclerosis who are severely disabled. I almost always find an excuse not to go to these meetings. When I do encounter severely disabled persons with MS, I find it very hard to relate to them. It is an intimation of my future which I am not ready to face. This "denial" can occur at the same time that a person is successfully adapting to the disease. The hallmark of an unsuccessful coping family is that they are ossified at the denial/resistant stage and do not make the necessary changes and accommodations to the disease; short-term "regression" to the denial mechanism can be normal and healthy as long as it does not interfere with the long-term adaptation that is necessary for accommodation to the disease process.

The couples most at risk are those who move through the coping process at very different rates. Couple stress is the strongest when one spouse is locked in denial while the other is already at the affirmation or adaptation stage. The psychological weight of the denying spouse is often more than the marriage can bear.

In the early stages of diagnosis, for example, the ill spouse, while willing to acknowledge the presence of the disease within the marriage, will sometimes pledge the well spouse to keep it a secret from family and friends. They preserve the fiction by pretending to others that, for example, "there is a back problem" to explain the reduced mobility. This often leaves the able-bodied spouse very lonely and constantly needing to be socially alert in order to maintain the lie. This conspiracy of silence often increases the marital tensions enormously because the well spouse needs to find some emotional support but cannot seek it—he or she must continue to preserve the fiction of a normally functioning family with a minor problem. The anger generated by this dilemma can be enormous. When these co-disabled spouses finally get to a support group, they often need ample time to unload all of the pent-up feelings of frustration and loneliness that such a situation imposes.

As I see it, there is no disease-specific coping mechanism. The responses to all of the diseases are pretty much the same. The psychological movement is always from denial to resistance to affirmation and finally to adaptation. With chronic, progressive disease, it is a continuous, open-ended process so that after the family has made an adaptation, they begin the process anew as the disease moves on. The process always demands a large amount of psychic energy. All spouses are most terrified by the dementing illness because it very rapidly changes the personality of the loved one. But, at some level, all of these diseases change the spouse's personality. It is the reaction to the disease as much as the disease itself. Someone who is in chronic pain or someone who is facing the loss of mobility or the loss of limbs or sight, is someone whose personality has changed. One can spend a lifetime wondering whether a mental change is due to the disease or to the reaction to the disease. In the long run, it doesn't matter. The focus of living for the ill person becomes so very different than for the well family members that this is no longer, nor will it ever be, the same person they knew prior to the diagnosis. The chronically ill are on a different course than anyone else in the family and it is the recognition of this that leads to the feelings of grief and the ever present feelings of loneliness that accompany all of the co-disabled.

My dictionary defines coping as "contending successfully with." All coping involves a stressful interaction between a person and his or her environment. Coping is any response to a difficult life situation that avoids or prevents distress. (Distress occurs when the individual experiences a great many demands with little or no control over them.) Coping also involves the possibility of growth and always demands change. The individual must come up with a new set of responses to contend with a changing set of either internal or external demands. Coping is a dynamic process and is not a stage, finally won and held forever. At times it is a moment-to-moment proposition.

With chronic, progressive illness, there are always new demands for coping because the illness is always changing; this demands flexibility because there is never any closure. It is a long, ever changing haul.

The advantage of gradual change in chronic illness is that you can make the life adjustment shifts in small increments, and even though obvious modifications feel like major shifts, a lot of subliminal change has taken place that leaves you better prepared to cope with the ultimate change than if you were dealing with a catastrophic change. Those people who have to undergo a catastrophic change do not have the luxury of the small alterations to prepare them. Change, however, is never easy because it always involves a letting go of some aspects of yourself: there can be no real growth without letting go of the old to assume the new. The stressor is what follows the letting go. In one sense, we are all underachieving, only giving as much to life and our living as is demanded of us; crisis is a means of forcing us to develop capacities and strengths that might otherwise lie dormant.

Oddly enough, coping becomes easier as the disability becomes more apparent. Chronic, progressive illness usually starts very slowly so that there is a relatively long period of time where the person looks normal and can pretend to others, if not to themselves, that there is nothing wrong. In all of these diseases, the patient looks so good for so long that everybody wonders if the illness might be psychosomatic. It is difficult to credit someone with being seriously ill when they look so well: it violates much of what we think we know about the disease. We are often apt to conclude that it must be in their mind. (My wife's neurologist, when he told us she had MS, said, "First of all, it is not in your head." I am eternally grateful to him for that.) It is thus difficult for other family members to accept the limitations imposed by the disease and they often conclude that the patient must be malingering; this often becomes a source of a great deal of anger. This is especially true for young children who equate diseases with bandages and looking sick. They become confused and angry when their parent can't do things because he or she is "sick" and yet looks normal.

Others in the family tend to overestimate the ill person's abilities (they are also practicing denial) and are confused and angered by the incompetencies that occasionally emerge. As the disability becomes more apparent, the views of others becomes more realistic, and much of the puzzled dismay of failed expectations disappears.

There are four general coping strategies.[12] The first and perhaps primary one is flight. Each individual, when confronted with a difficult and potentially stressful situation, has to decide whether to fight or flee. At times it is very appropriate to run; there are life situations with which you are unable to cope and flight is the best alternative. Often, however, it is the perception of inadequacy that can trigger flight. As long as you feel totally overwhelmed, flight is the most likely response, either that or denial which is a psychological flight. Fleeing, however, always leaves you vulnerable to guilt and a loss of self-esteem. In addition to the actual flight, as in a divorce, there is the psychological flight that almost all spouses experience, varying from a feeling of separation that is experienced as unreality, to the emotional detachment often experienced, as in the fantasies of your own death or the death of your spouse. (Figuratively, the spouse is dying.) The latter fantasy, of course, would be the ultimate release from a painful situation. Fantasies about a spouse's death are common; it is difficult for many spouses to admit that they dream and think about their spouse dying (I frequently do). This "death wish" is in part due to wanting to make the problem go away—not the spouse necessarily, but the stress of the disease. It is the "ultimate" solution to a difficult and painful problem and, as such, it is quite normal; although it often generates enormous amounts of guilt.

When psychologists rate life situations for stress, they usually put death of a spouse and/or divorce as the most stressful. My own particular view is that living with someone who is chronically and progressively ill is eventually more stressful than either death or divorce. With death or divorce, there is a termination and the surviving spouses can make a permanent adjustment to the painful situation and go on with their lives; with chronic, progressive disability, the well spouse is constantly being forced to make new adjustments and is almost always living in a state of anxiety; the stress is continuous.

The death fantasies also may be helpful in preparing for the actual death of the spouse: it is referred to as anticipatory mourning. It is a psychologically protective process that enables the spouse to cope with the actual death more constructively than if the event was not anticipated—it is sometimes a dress rehearsal.

If the person decides to stay in the difficult situation, the next strategy employed is to try to modify the environment. The diseases presented in this book are not amenable to a cure but many of the ramifications of the diseases can be controlled. Thus, a wheelchair can make life easier for the physically disabled, medication can reduce some of the pain of arthritis and lupus, and joint replacement in some cases can alleviate some of the crippling effects of arthritis. Drugs can modify some of the effects of Alzheimer's disease and insulin can control many of the symptoms of diabetes. The trick in trying to modify the stressful situation is in knowing what can be modified and doing it, and then learning to accept what cannot be changed—not always easy to do; to err is to be frustrated.

The third strategy for reducing stress is to change the way we look at the situation. This is known as cognitively neutralizing the stressor. It is always the cognitive process that determines the emotional intensity of any event. Events have meaning in direct proportion to how we choose to see them. Probably the most frequently used cognitive strategy is to say "It could be worse" as in "He could have cancer." This is used a great deal by family and friends who are trying to make you feel better. After they say it could be worse, they set about trying to find someone, someplace, who is in more difficulty than you are (it usually is not very hard to do). When someone tries to "help" us in this way, Cari usually forestalls the whole thing by responding "Yes, and it could be better, too." The problem with using positive comparisons is that no matter how bad something else might be, there are still going to be times when you do feel bad; (there is much for us to feel bad about). When that happens, you are prone to feeling guilty as though you had no right to feel grief. Using positive comparisons often buys some short-term psychological relief but the pain of the disability will always intrude; the effectiveness of looking for someone worse off than you begins to fade quickly. There are other more fruitful ways of reframing perceptions which will be discussed later.

The fourth strategy is to deal directly with the stress. No matter how successful fantasies, modification, and using cognitive neutralizers may be, there will always be stress. This can be dealt with directly by finding activities that reduce stress. These can range from the mundane, such as biting fingernails, to the exotic, such as hiking in the Himalayas. Some of the stress reducers reported to me in my interviews with families have been: baking pies, meditation, yoga, gardening, hot baths, music, aerobic dancing, and family activities (Grandchildren are great for this). Almost all effective strategies involve a time-out experience—there has to be time away from the chronically ill family member. For the shadow spouses, there is so little that they can control about the disease and the spouses' reaction to the disease, that they invariably seek those activities that can provide them with some control. Gardening for me has that quality; as the song goes, when you plant a radish seed, you get a radish. There is a predictability and control in gardening that I find attractive. What is effective for one person may not work for another, but the stress reducers that do seem almost universally effective are exercise, and perhaps almost equally universal in application is work. In fact, one can almost define the co-disabled spouse as someone who looks forward to going to work and dreads going home.

For me, work has been a lifesaver. (Writing this book has also been a big help.) Whenever I leave on a business trip, it is always with mixed feelings composed of equal parts of guilt that I am leaving and my wife is staying, worry that she may not be able to take care of herself, and relief that I can move freely without having to consider her needs. The trips for me become a societally sanctioned form of escape. I also understand now why geniuses such as Mozart and Beethoven could produce such beautiful pieces of music while their personal lives were in such shambles. The energy that would have gone into their interpersonal relationships went into their music. You can escape into your work. I have been professionally productive (not that I'm a genius) since Cari's illness. I have also produced a lovely garden.

Escape is not the only reason for the increased work. Sometimes it is a function of the economics of the situation. Wives often have to go to work in order to support the family, and husbands have to increase their work in order to support the larger financial demands that are now placed on their family because of the disease. There is also the possibility that the spouse may have to take an early retirement from work in order to nurse the husband or wife, and there is a strong need to increase their savings in order to support them both in retirement.

The increased intensity given to work also comes about as a result of the co-disabled person's recognition of their own vulnerability and mortality. When disease strikes someone close to you, it is a reminder that it could and might happen to you; you get intimidations of your own morality. What happens is that you want to get as much as possible out of life and get it in while you can. You are much less apt to postpone events because you recognize that you may never have this opportunity again. There is an intensity to the living and to working. One sees this frequently in the shadow spouse.

Exercise also has almost universal applicability as a stress reducer, in part because it always a time-out experience that gets the person away from confronting the disabled spouse. It also serves to have an emotionally calming effect; repetitive exercise such as jogging, swimming, or bicycling puts the mind into a meditative state. When I start out on my morning jog emotionally upset, I am almost always able to return much calmer. Somehow the "problems" seem to work out, and jogging for me is almost a moving mediation that I know is vital to both my mental and physical well being. Also, by keeping myself in good physical shape, I seem more capable of dealing better with emotional stress, than when I am not in good physical shape.

These, then, are the four strategies of coping: flight, environmental modification, cognitive neutralization, and direct stress reduction. Individuals can and do use any and all of these strategies in order to come to grips with difficult life situations.

Following are some ideas about coping culled mainly from my own experiences:

Changing the Household

Disability is always a matter of context and all handicaps are situation specific. In a marvelous short story, "Country of the Blind," H. G. Wells tells a story of a sighted man who stumbles upon a lost community in which everyone is blind. He becomes convinced that with his sight they will make him King, as he keeps saying "In the valley of the blind, the one eyed man will be King." To his dismay, he discovers that his vision is a disadvantage. The community has no lighting; they work at night and have no use for sight in any of their interactions. In fact, they are concerned as to why he seems so handicapped. The theme of this story is that "handicap" is always a function of context. Disability is a reduced function: handicap is related to environmental barriers that in many cases can be removed or modified so as to minimize the effects of the disability on a person's functioning. As Cari and I have bought appliances and modified our home we have reduced the effects of her disability. Without them she would be pretty much bed and house bound now and thus very "handicapped."

With a disabled spouse, one must make the necessary changes in the environment in order to minimize the handicap. The paradox of this is that as we actually get each device or modification, which does make life easier for us, the disability becomes more evident and it is always a psychologically painful time when we must acknowledge the loss by the need for the new appliance or modification.

We have also been making changes in our household management as Cari has to give up some of her former responsibilities. I have taken on some of them —I now do all of the shopping and most of the cooking. What I have to be sure about is that I do not overload myself and here is where friends, family, and purchased services come to the fore. Cari has marshalled women from her Temple's sisterhood as well as friends and neighbors in organizing a rotation of volunteers to come each day to help her exercise. I don't know if this does any good in terms of arresting the MS but it boosts Cari's morale and provides social stimulation. In addition, it provides me with support that I need. I go to work knowing that someone is going to come into the house. Debbie, our next door neighbor, makes our bed and waters our plants whenever I am out of town, and as I tell her frequently, "If you don't make it as a lawyer, you can always make it as a chambermaid." Neighbors will, without asking, clear our walks with their snowblowers. My children have also been helpful although now that they live far away and are deeply emersed in their own lives they cannot help as much as they would like.

The research on Alzheimer's disease[13] has shown that successful coping is a function of the caregiver's health and unpaid help; we have been fortunate to have both.

We are also, at Cari's urging, purchasing services. We now have our home cleaned and we have even begun talking about the possibility of hiring a home health aide for a few hours in the afternoon to help Cari prepare dinner.

In some ways the physical changes are easier to make than the service changes. Removing architectural barriers at this point increases mobility and gives me more of a spouse. Purchasing services from others makes the loss of spouse seem more obvious. At some level, a spouse is never truly replaceable.

Participating in Alternative Activities

The disability mandates a change in lifestyle. We can no longer hike and run together as we used to. We don't share in as many outside activities as we formerly did. I think twice before we go any place because of the stress of getting her in and out and consequently we just do not go out as often as we formerly did. To try to recapture the past by trying to engage in the same activities we used to do is always a loss. We must acknowledge and mourn the loss of that other life and then go on from there.

In place of the hiking and running, we have found some alternate activities. We rediscovered the joy of listening to the radio. (Prairie Home Companion is a particular favorite of ours.) Reading aloud to one another, watching old movies on our VCR, and entertaining intimate friends over small luncheons and dinners are other shared pleasures. A big date for us is to buy take-out food and a movie. I also invariably buy Cari's favorite candy which enables me to deliver my famous line "Nobody knows the Truffles I've seen." (After a while it begins to wear thin.) We also now do most of our shopping through catalogues (although one of the hidden costs of disability is that you don't always have the resources to shop comparatively to take advantage of sales).

Our new life is not better or worse than our old one; it is just different. I have found that it doesn't matter what we do together so much as the quality of the doing. I have also found that I can continue to do some of the things that give me satisfaction with people other than my wife so that in some ways my life is much richer now for these new-found activities.

Helping

Probably the most difficult issue for the caregiver spouse to deal with is how much help to give. It is so easy and at times so tempting to do things yourself and bypass the spouse's fumbling efforts to do them that one can so easily rob an ailing spouse of dignity, and in subtle ways undermine confidence in his or her ability to cope with the environment. One can very easily create a dependent spouse much sooner than is necessary; this is known as learned helplessness, and on the caretaker's part, as dysfunctional helping.

The rule Cari and I have evolved over the years is that she gets no help unless she asks for it. It is sometimes very hard for me to follow this rule, as when I hear a crash in another room followed by cursing. I steel myself not to go rushing to the rescue or even ask, "What happened?" I clench my teeth and wait for her to ask for help. If she does, I give it without hesitation. This rule has clarified our relationship and our communication. It has made life easier for us.

Cari often remarks that she is so tired of having to be grateful that I often try to anticipate her needs so that she doesn't have to ask. It is a very thin line I tread between being truly helpful and not diminishing her self-esteem and confidence by overhelping. We don't have much of a margin with which to operate.

What I probably have the most difficulty doing is letting her help me. This comes out of my own fear that she might hurt herself or break something. Yet she is still quite capable of doing many things and it becomes so invalidating of her as a viable human being not to permit her to help me. I have to constantly guard against diminishing her with my physical competence and recognize her equality and respect her dignity as a person.

Not Owning the Disease

Although I am a co-disabled spouse, I need to keep reminding myself that I don't have multiple sclerosis; Cari does. By this I mean that the primary responsibility for managing the course of the disease is hers and not mine. We invariably get into trouble when I step over that equator of responsibility. When I go on trips, for example, I used to arrange for my children or neighbors to "visit," ostensibly it was to walk the dog, in reality it was to check that Cari was not in trouble. This was to assuage my guilt and anxiety about leaving her alone. My wife saw through the subterfuge and resented my lack of trust in her ability to manage for herself. Now, when I have a business trip, I just give my wife enough warning and ask her what she wants to do. I no longer arrange for "wife sitters"; this is her problem: besides the dog has died. In a similar vein I do not make decisions regarding the course of treatment. Cari has been offered the possibility of taking cytoxan (she refused) and other experimental drugs to try to arrest the course of MS. She instead has opted for more alternative treatments mainly diet, meditation, and exercise. I have supported her in all of her decisions. I generally go with her to all important doctor visits and serve mainly as a sounding board for her decisions. Cari has also taken full responsibility for her doctor's appointments as well as doing all the hard research on any new appliance or device to increase her functioning. Without her taking this responsibility I don't think we could have survived.

Altering the Perspective

Disability is always in the eye of the beholder. We can have either a problem or a challenge. It is all in how we choose to look at situations. It doesn't feel as though there is a choice in the perception of events, but it is there nonetheless. We give meaning to the events in our lives and we can see an event any way we choose to. Early on in the course of this disease, Cari fell in the parking lot of the supermarket and had to be helped up by a passerby. She came home devastated that here was one more piece of evidence of her increasing weakness and disability. I listened to her pain and then I commented that she must have made that man's day. He must have gone home feeling good about himself. We talked at length about that and concluded that she is now a walking "mitzvah." (Mitzvah is a Yiddish word meaning doing good without any thought of gain.) Although Cari would prefer not to be the one helped all the time, if we were all helpers, there would be nobody to help; so to be rabbinical about this, it is also a mitzvah to let someone else do a mitzvah.

Now as she scoots around town in her motorized wheelchair trying to lead a "normal life," she is often told she has become other people's inspiration. At times she would like another role but if this is what we must be, so be it. So in addition to living with a moving mitzvah I live with a rolling inspiration: this is not easy.

For myself, I have had to redefine "giving." In a child/adult book *The Giving Tree*,[14] Shel Silverstein has written a story about a needy boy who keeps coming to a tree to ask for things he wants. The tree unhesitatingly gives him parts of himself until at the end he is reduced to the barest stump. The story has always disturbed me as I think it is the wrong concept of giving. Giving should not diminish, it should expand. There is a lot of getting in giving. In fact I have decided for myself that I don't give. When I do something for someone else (for example, my wife), it is because it enhances me and the recipient of my largess is under no obligation to me. I should thank her for giving me that chance to feel good about myself; my wife owes me nothing. Keeping this perception of giving in mind avoids, for me, the resentment that one finds in many co-disabled spouses because of the increased demands on their time and energy.

I know that each day I wake up choosing to stay in the marriage, and knowing that I have that choice keeps me here. And with that choice comes the responsibility of making that choice work the best way I can.

Accepting the Pain

One lesson I have had to learn and one that I keep having to relearn is that it is not my job to make Cari feel better. She is generally an "up" person and I think this is why people are so willing to help her, but from time to time this disease really gets her down (me too) and she tells me how bad she feels. My role used to be to try to make her feel better by rationally trying to solve the "problem" or if that did not work by distracting her from the pain. As I keep finding out, these strategies do not work. All they seem to do is invalidate her feelings and the best thing I can do is just listen to her. Listening often seems so passive to me that the role of listener is a hard one for me to accept. I still have a strong urge to fix it. Cari has taught me that all she wants at these times is an empathetic ear and I am constantly learning that listening is the best thing I can do. Cari helps me now by prefacing her statements with "All I want to do is tell you how I feel." This has made a big difference for us.

Seeking an Explanation

Everyone involved with chronic illness that has no known cause must wrestle with the difficult question, "Why me?" It's so easy to feel picked on, as though you are one of life's bull's eyes for misery. It is a tough question because it leads to a fundamental evaluation of why we are here and what our purpose is in life and living. This question always leads to an existential crisis about the meaning of life, sometimes of very monumental proportions. Beyond the pain of the disease many people have to redefine their existence and their relationship to God. Most people believe that God punishes evil and rewards good. If something bad befalls you, either you were bad or God is bad; a very uncomfortable dilemma. Many deeply religious people have adopted a frequently used explanation, saying that God has some purpose in giving their family illness to deal with and even though they can't divine a reason for it, they still trust Him. Here are some explanations of co-disabled spouses that I have interviewed:

> I think the thing that helps me cope the most is my spiritual faith, because I know without a doubt that there is a reason and a purpose for all of this. I don't feel God has made it happen; I think the Lord knew it did happen. I think he has allowed it to happen. I don't know why yet. That was one of my first questions when we got the diagnosis. Why is this happening? But you know I've seen Henry's attitude on life change, especially over the last couple of years. He's very sympathetic towards other people with a handicap. Very understanding about women. I think in school, he's become more understanding with the kids. He really works with a bunch of bandits. It's a tough school. And when the girls find themselves pregnant, even before his own daughter, he was the one they went to for counseling. He always gives everybody a fair shake. He's more compassionate. And myself, I was never aware of handicap accessibility to a building but I am now. You know, I see places where he could not go just because he couldn't open a door and if he ends up in a wheelchair in a year or so, he's going to be really cut off even more. So that's something I'm more aware of. It's made our kids a lot more sensitive not just to their father—just to us as parents. They have become very sensitive kids. My middle daughter graduates this year and she wants to be a social worker and it's had a big impact on how she looks at people—not to just dismiss it.

Another spouse said:

> There was a period of time in the early years when I didn't

cope very well. I come from a very religious background and had a very strong personal faith and at one time it wasn't enough to hold me. I studied astrology like mad! I was hoping to determine what the future would be. And then I knew it was wrong. It was really a stupid thing! I have reconciled this as a Christian by believing that God allows us to partake of all these problems—that nobody escapes. We are a part of life and He is not going to save the physical body and I believe in the life hereafter. I believe our spirits are sound. I believe that God's purpose works out and that his purpose is just totally different than ours.

And yet another spouse had this to say:

I can't see any good in this disease. I cannot understand almighty God's thinking. We think like human beings, we can't think like the Almighty so we can't know but to have faith, and I have to pray for that faith constantly because it's tested. It's tested constantly. I haven't gotten angry. I don't understand myself why I haven't got angry. I don't know how this happened. He was a good living man who always lived a good, clean life. I just pray it's not heredity. I think sometimes it might have been better if we were old in the sense of 80. Maybe it would have been worse. I couldn't have cared for him. I wouldn't have had the strength that I have at this age. Yet we would have had all those in-between years to enjoy each other. There's no good answer. No matter what you go through in your life, your hell is the worst hell you can see; this is hell. This is hell. There are no glorious answers. There are none. There is no reason, there is no rhyme.

Another frequently heard response is that "God only gives you what you can handle." So if I were weaker, my wife wouldn't have MS? As you can tell this one doesn't work very well with me.

Other co-disabled people vent their anger at God and refuse to go back to church. These people often stay stuck in their anger and bitterness. One cognitive reframing that prevents me from getting stuck in the "Why me?" is the "Why not me?" response. What is so special about me that something bad couldn't happen? Who ever promised me that I wouldn't have a wife with MS? And as my wife says often, "Whom would we wish it on?"

Cari often recounts a tale of a women whose son died and who went to the Bhudda requesting that her son be brought back to life. The Bhudda told her, "Go to the village and collect a mustard seed from each house that has not experienced some loss. If you can collect three seeds, I will bring your son back to life." The woman knocked on every door in the village and could not get one seed.

Loss is part of life and if we live long enough we all experience loss. Some of us experience loss earlier in our lives but loss is the price we pay for life. I refer again to the R. L. Stevenson quote at the beginning of this book that says that life is often a matter of playing a poor hand well. Multiple sclerosis is the hand my wife and I were dealt, and somehow I feel we must make good things happen from it, by playing this "hand" as well as we can.

Some families that I've met take an entirely pragmatic view and cease to worry about an explanation, trying to cope with the problem (or challenge if you will) at hand, dealing with it on a one-day-at-a-time basis. To a certain extent, any successfully coping couple must deal with the disease on a day-to-day basis. To look ahead too far is to be engulfed in fear and anxiety; and to look back is to have guilt and despair. The present offers us our possibilities. I have learned to take it one-day-at-a-time and if that's too long, as it is on some days, one-hour-at-a-time. There are some days when I am reduced to minutes. When all is said and done the only really meaningful question is "Where do I go from here?"

Seeking a Cure

The lack of a medically recognized cure for any of the diseases described in this book has given rise to a host of questionable "cures." These range from snake venom to exotic diets with countless other choices in between. It is possible to spend a lifetime running from one treatment to another, and I have met people who have tried everything in their desperation. Cure seeking can be a distraction from dealing with the problem at hand and, in the long run, is not a very fruitful use of energy. This is not to say that one does not or should not keep alert to potential cures and hope and pray for one. One must learn to accept without being resigned. But for me, searching for the cure needs to be on a back burner; my prayer is not so much for a cure as it is that the disease process be arrested. I cannot afford to spend much of my psychic or physical energy on seeking. I have so much to do now and only so much energy to spend—I would rather spend it on making the most of what I have.

I need to develop the wisdom to know the difference between what I can and cannot do, and find the strength and determination to accomplish what is doable. I need also the maturity to accept what is no longer possible. The hardest lesson for me to learn in life is that there are problems that I cannot solve.

Keeping it in Perspective

Cari, quite rightly, insists that I never refer to her as an "MS victim." She insists that she is more than her disability, that her ability to walk or not is just part of her. I have to see that too. There are times and days when I feel like I am drowning in multiple sclerosis. It seems to dominate all of our conversation and our life. When we can get it into perspective, it becomes a feature of our lives to be dealt with in the same way we must consider our aging and our choices in living and working. We all need time out from the disease. I look forward to days when the word MS is not spoken in the house. And if only for one moment and time, we can pretend that we are like every other family that is okay.

Managing the Changes

Change is inevitable in life, and we cannot hold it back. In fact, if we do not anticipate change, we usually get overwhelmed by it. Change, though, is frightening because it presents new and different demands and, unless we are confident in our ability to cope with events, we resist the change. Change, however, is never easy because it always involves a letting go of some aspect of ourselves. The truth of the matter is that all families and the people in them are organisms in a continuous process of changing while trying to remain the same. We can mourn the structure that was lost but it makes more sense to look at the possibilities of the new.

I have also learned not to second-guess myself. When confronted with a need to make a change, I marshall as many facts as I can and then move ahead with the decision. Sometimes the decisions I've made have not always turned out to be the most fruitful and then I change them. These are really not mistakes since they invariably provide me with new, valuable information. It's only a mistake if I do it a second time. To allow myself to wallow in "should haves" is self-defeating. It limits my ability or willingness to make future decisions. There are no blueprints laid out for me in this business, and we often must make it up as we go along. Cari and I are a unique experiment of one, and while we can and do find the experience of others useful, the ultimate responsibility is ours, and I need to feel that we have made the best decision for us on the best available information at that time. I also find that I cannot and should not plan more than one year ahead. That seems to be the most manageable time frame for me. Things change rapidly and I need to be flexible to the change. Looking too far ahead is also too frightening.

Seeking Emotional Support

Any catastrophic event that changes our status isolates us from the familiar. To have a chronically ill spouse often means that we may not be able to get emotional support from persons we formerly went to for help. Nobody quite understands and can really empathize with what the families are going through unless they have been there themselves. Try as they might, relatives and friends rarely can give the emotional support that is needed. They sympathize, rather than empathize, and in some instances, they take on the pain. Thus, the disabled couple often become reluctant to share with them for fear of burdening them further and thus isolating themselves even more. (This is especially true of parents.)

The place where I can obtain the most emotional support and understanding is with other spouses of chronically ill people. The support groups have been one place that I have most often found the emotional sustenance I need. I have also had to learn that it is okay to ask for help. I have had to change my notions of strength and self sufficiency. I know that I can be (and am) a strong person who, at times, needs help and, at times, cries. I used to be, and to a certain extent still am, the kind of person who, when lost, never asks for directions, but I have loosened up some with that as I recognize that the truly strong person is one who can ask for help and lets himself appear "weak" in other people's eyes. (That is also the gift we give to others by letting them help us.)

Nuland[3] caught the support group notion very well when he wrote:

> In the case of Alzheimer's disease, it is rarely the patient who recognizes the need for company in the journey through travail. But there is probably no disability of our time in which the presence of support groups can help so decisively to ensure the emotional survival of the closest witness to the disintegration . . . They function not only to provide help but also as advocates of increased funding for research and clinical improvements. There is strength in numbers, even when the numbers are only one or two understanding people who can soften the anguish by the simple act of listening (p. 106).

For the past several years I have been facilitating spouse support groups for the local chapter of the MS society. I have found the best format for the group (and for me) is four 2-hour meetings stretched over two weeks. I have found that trying to hold more than four meetings is counter productive as the well family members are usually so strapped for time that many can barely make the four sessions. Also many do drop out. Usually the first session is a highly cathartic one, because seldom are well spouses given a chance or a format to express their feelings. The feelings are so pent up that they start spilling as each participant gets a chance to tell his or her story and once the dam is breached the flood commences. Some members of the group are frightened by the outright display of emotion and they do not return for subsequent groups. Many of them do come back at another time when they are more psychologically prepared to deal with the emotional aspects of chronic illness. I do not screen the participants for the level of disability of their spouse. So in the group there may be participants who are just embarking on the progressive disability route and others who are near the end of their journey with a very disabled spouse. This disability disparity is often unsettling to the newly diagnosed and they are not ready to confront such a scenario for themselves. In one of the first groups I facilitated one man asked if anyone knew what constituted a signature as his wife could barely make an "X". That scared the hell out of me and I wanted to leave too.

I have also found that the intensity of the well spouse's feelings is not necessarily related to the degree of disability in their husband or wife. There are several factors involved in the willingness to display feelings. One is obviously culturally related to how much talking about feelings is part of the person's upbringing and experience. The other factor is how much communication the well spouse has with other people. There is no doubt in my mind that the angriest and most frustrated participants are the ones who have pledged to "keep MS a secret." They are just so clammed up with their feeling that once they get to the group it does not take much to unleash the flood of emotions: sometimes burying the more emotionally inhibited participants in such frightening scenarios that they do not continue in the group.

After the initial cathartic experience, the remaining group usually settles into a more relaxed format as each individual further refines his or her story and begins to share solutions to the problem of living with someone with MS. Intimacy usually happens quickly as there is the almost instant recognition of a fellow traveler on a singular journey and loneliness, if only for a while, is alleviated.

If there is any wisdom in this chapter, it is due to my participation in these groups for the past ten years and this writing is compiled from many people's different experiences. I owe my fellow travelers much.

Taking Care of Oneself

Leadership, at least as defined in some circles, is what you've got left over after you take care of yourself. I have to constantly remind myself of that simple truth. If I am going to be doing a lot of "giving" in this relationship, I have to be doing a lot of getting somewhere else or there will be nothing to give. The truth of the matter is that I am the most important member of our family, because if I go under, our family will no longer be able to function.

I often feel guilty when I do something that I feel that I need to do for myself and that my wife can't share. Even though Cari urges me to go and do (she recognizes the need, perhaps more deeply than I do, to take care of myself and often says, "If I can't, does it mean that you shouldn't?"), I still feel the guilt. I have learned to acknowledge the feeling and still behave in a way that is in our best interests.

I often feel reluctant to go, and then I think, "How can it possibly be helpful to her if I got sick, or badly out of shape because I gave up running or I was unhappy and resentful?" It could become very easy for me to make a disabled person of myself. I have learned to be, and am, always it seems, in the process of relearning how important it is that I take care of my needs first. For me, a powerful metaphor for this occurs every time I fly. The stewardess explains that if the oxygen mask should be needed in flight and you are travelling with a child, to put the mask on your face first. I always have to remind myself of this when I do something good for myself and put my needs first. Of course this mandates that I not confuse my needs with my wants, and at times, I have to be willing to postpone the satisfaction of my wants because someone else's needs are more pressing.

There is also the need for periodic time outs—coping with a loved one who has chronic, progressive illness is like running a marathon; you are in for the long haul. I remember reading an article by a writer who was in the lead truck watching Bill Rogers set, at that time, the record for the Boston Marathon. Rogers, who was far ahead of the field stopped (which is unheard of in marathoning circles) had a drink and looked around. At another point he stopped and retied his shoelace and still went on to set a record pace for the distance. The writer at first thought that if he hadn't stopped twice, he would have broken the record even further and then, after considering it for a moment realized maybe he had set the record because he had stopped. So, too, with the co-disabled; if we want to finish the race, perhaps not in record time but to finish it, we must stop every so often and take a break for ourselves.

A shadow wife describes how she takes care of herself psychologically:

> I also try in my mind to maintain that distance that is needed to keep it a healthy relationship because I know that the facts are there and I could easily be without him one day. And I keep thinking, "Well, what would I do?" I've got things planned out. I have projects like you wouldn't believe. I'll write books, I'm into painting, I have my sewing, I've got my crafts. We are antiquers. I have this thing in my mind about building a house and selling it and building another house and selling it. I love that sort of thing. The possibilities are endless. I'd just love to be my own person. I keep saying to myself, we've got it good now but I'm going to keep looking forward to the future.

Another thing that has helped me has been trying to adhere to "Ten Commandments" written by 90-year-old Elodie Armstrong who had multiple sclerosis for forty years. I culled this from an Ann Landers column.

1) Thou shalt not worry, for worry is the most unproductive of all human activities.

2) Thou shalt not be fearful, for most of the things we fear never come to pass.

3) Though shalt not cross bridges before you get to them, for no one yet has succeeded in accomplishing this.

4) Thou shalt face each problem as it comes. You can handle only one at a time anyway.

5) Thou shalt not take problems to bed with you for they make very poor bedfellows.

6) Thou shalt not borrow other people's prolems; they can take better care of them than you can.

7) Thou shalt not try to relive yesterday for good or ill—it is gone. Concentrate on what is happening in your life today.

8) Thou shalt count thy blessings, never over looking the small ones, for a lot of small blessings add up to a big one.

9) Thou shalt be a good listener, for only when you listen do you hear ideas different from your own. It's very hard to learn something new when you're talking.

10) Thou shalt not become bogged down by frustration, for 90 percent of it is rooted in self pity and it will only interfere with positive action.

As a summary of this chapter here are Luterman's ten rules for living with a chronically ill person:

1) Take good care of yourself. You are the most important family member. If you get ill, your family collapses. Time-outs to restore your perspective and to maintain your own health are absolutely essential. The two almost universal coping strategies that are successfully used are work and exercise. Don't let yourself get overtired - you cope much better when you are rested.

2) Give yourself periodic time-outs at home; negotiate with your spouse to have times during the day when he or she is not permitted to ask you to do anything. These times need to be followed by periods when you will do anything needed, no questions asked.

3) Be careful of over helping. You can easily create a dependent spouse by teaching learned helplessness. The best rule of thumb is to give help only when asked. At other times, anticipate needs and give the help without seeming to.

4) Make changes in the household as needed. Do not go too far out in your time frame. A short-term focus of 6-12 months is desirable. Psychologically, it is sometimes necessary to do this on a day-to-day basis and if that is too long, try moment-to-moment.

5) Don't mourn for long the things lost. Stay focused on what you have. Develop alternative activities; for example, substitue reading aloud to each other for the hiking you have lost.

6) Don't own the disease. While you are profoundly affected by the disease, you don't

have it. Unless your spouse is mentally incompetent, the day-to-day management of the disease is his or her responsibility, not yours.

7) Do not be afraid to ask for help. Do not expect other people to read your mind. Remember that the most successful coping well spouses are the ones whose health is good and who have a great deal of unpaid support. Do not feel diffident about asking for help from friends and family.

8) Keep the disease in perspective. You and your spouse are more than a disease—this is just one feature of your life, albeit an important one. It is okay to spend time not thinking or talking about the disease.

9) Seek emotional support. The most likely place is a group of fellow well spouses. Find within your contacts individuals who can listen to your pain without helping you to feel guilty. They are rare to find—when you do so, hang on to them. Remember, you have a serious problem and you are entitled to your pain.

10) Disability is a matter of how you look at it. Chronic illness can be seen as a terrible tragedy in your life or as the powerful teacher that it is. We do not know why it has entered our lives, but it is there nonetheless. Remember the quote of Robert Louis Stevenson that says, "Life is not a matter of holding good cards, but of playing a poor hand well." The challenge to you is to play this lousy "hand" you have been dealt very well.

Reading the following piece, author unknown, has helped me a great deal:

TO LET GO

To Let Go is not to stop caring,
It's recognizing I can't do it for someone else.
To Let Go is not to cut myself off,
It's realizing I can't control another.

To Let go is not to enable,
But to allow learning from natural consequences.
To Let Go is not to fight powerlessness,
But to accept that the outcome is not in my hands.

To Let Go is not to try to change or blame others,
It's to make the most of myself.
To Let Go is not to care for, it's to care about.
To Let Go is not to fix, it's to be supportive.

To Let Go is not to judge,
It's to allow another to be a human being.
To Let Go is not to try to arrange outcomes,
But to allow others to affect their own destinies.

To Let Go is not to be protective,
It's to permit another to face their own reality.
To Let Go is not to regulate anyone,
But to strive to become what I can be.

To Let Go is not to fear less, it's to love more.

CHAPTER 6

The Good Of It All

As I write this chapter I am reminded of a W. Somerset Maugham anecdote. The author was feted on the occasion of his 80th birthday and was asked to contribute some closing remarks. He began by saying "There are many advantages to being 80 years of age." Then there followed a very long pause during which his audience became very uncomfortable. "Only I can't think of any" he finally continued to the relief of everyone. He then sat down, to thunderous applause and laughter.

In writing this chapter I want to see the positives in MS before sitting down and I do think there are some things to be grateful for.

I don't want to be a pollyanna but my mental health and my ability to cope successfully with the very difficult situation of living with someone who has chronic, progress illness is based on three cardinal rules. One, that I accept my feelings for what they are and only judge my behavior, second, that I stay with a short-term focus, and third, that I look at what I have gained rather than what I have lost.

Here is what I have gained:

1) *Rearrangement of Priorities*

For me, a lot of the pettiness of living has dropped away. I have learned, I think, what is important and things that I previously worried about, such as my appearance or material goods, seem so trivial now. It's always hard to tease out what changes are due to the MS in my wife, and what would have occurred as part of my natural, maturing evolution into adulthood. I have attained a clear sense of what is important and I seldom feel as though I am wasting time. I have become immensely more productive in my work because I recognize how time-limited I am and how fragile my world is. I think I have gained a deeper appreciation of *being* as more important than *accomplishing*. I have also learned to take more risks in my life—realizing how fragile it all is anyway—and no matter how cautious you are and how good you are, bad things can happen to you. Fear, if I allow it to be, can be a very restricting emotion; it will narrow my options and limit my opportunities. It can imprison me in a world full of dangers and restrict me from seeing all the possibilities of life. To be alive after all is to be at risk. In fact one can over-balance in life by caution, when you try to ride a bicycle too slowly, you invariably fall. For me and my wife, the fall has already happened—so what the hell! In an existential sense, life itself is a fatal illness.

Probably the saddest man I have met was a spouse in his 60s whose wife of a similar age had been stricken with a rapid, progressive form of multiple sclerosis and was now bedridden. He kept lamenting how they had saved all their lives to spend their "golden years" traveling and now they couldn't go anywhere. I've learned that these are my golden years and my wife and I seldom put off anything. We do what we want when we can. This is not to say we don't save or plan for the future, but we know that the future is very uncertain and cloudy, and we are inclined to do it now. Our living and the fun of living has intensified. I am never bored. I know I have only a limited time to do things. There is a recognition of my own vulnerability so that there is an increased intensity in what I do. I want to use the limited time I have fully.

One bonus of MS is seen in the room we built on our house. It is quite large and sunny with a skylight and a large picture window overlooking the garden. We both can experience the changing of the seasons and the growth of the plants. In all likelihood we would not have built this room if it were not for the MS. We also have, adjoining the room, a large handicapped accessible bathroom with a roll-in shower. I sometimes think that if I became disabled it would be useful for me too. I guess in one sense we are all only temporarily able-bodied. Awareness of this has led me to appreciate my body and its ability to move. I try to take good care of it.

2) *A Deeper Marital Commitment and Communication*

In our generation, a husband and wife were expected to have definite role responsibilities, and even though Cari was always a working wife, she would come home and work as well. I would often help, but the primary responsibilities for the home were hers. Now our marriage is much more of a cooperative working marriage, albeit somewhat overbalanced on my end. I am really involved in this marriage in ways that I wasn't before.

Our level of communication has also deepened since the diagnosis of MS. We are more inclined to discuss feelings and any issues that are disturbing either one of us. I think that there has been both an explicit and implicit recognition that openness in our communication is an absolute requirement for our remaining married. The stress of the disease has forced us to adopt rules for our living together that intensify our bonds; for example, we don't go to bed angry and always try to keep anger out of the bedroom. It is not easy to do and there are evenings we have sat up working things out. It would be so easy for us to live alone together if we are not careful. The stress and strain is there but also present is the love and caring.

3) *Increased Compassion*

I have always worked in the helping professions, as both a teacher and a clinician working with hearing-impaired people and with the parents of young deaf children in particular. I think that my initial work was as much intellectual as it was emotional. I find now my relationships are much more emotionally intense. I am more inclined to display my feelings with everyone. I find I cry now much more readily than I ever had before. I feel within me a softness and caring that I had not discovered before my wife's illness. Rabbi Kushner, whose son died at age 14, had this to say about disaster:[15]

> It teaches you something about your strengths and acquaints you with your limitations. If I had not gone through the experience of my son's illness and death, I'm sure I would have had a much more intellectual, less compassionate approach to other people's misfortunes. It was a high price to pay but it has made me a much deeper, more helpful person that I would have been otherwise.

4) *Increased Friends*

Chronic illness has a way of bringing out in others that which most makes us human: the capacity to care. All the help and outpouring of care and concern from others that we have received does not allow me to be cynical about the human race. Because of the MS, Cari and I have met many wonderful people who have given so readily of themselves and who have become our friends. We feel very fortunate. It is also a built in Litmus test whereby we can determine who are our true friends; we have discarded former friends who no longer call.

5) *A Renewed Sense of Direction and Purpose in Life*

For many healthy spouses, the disability in their partner has increased their sense of personal worth. They now know that they are needed, and although at times that can seem overwhelming, it also feels good. There is now a direction and purpose in life: they are focused.

The role reversal that occurs in many marriages when the husband is the one who is disabled enables the woman to discover this strength that might never have been uncovered if not for the illness. Many spouses find a new vocation for themselves. I have yet to meet a wheelchair salesperson who wasn't also a co-disabled spouse. This is often true of the children of disability who often enter a helping profession.

It is not uncommon to find couples with chronic illness becoming active in helping to alleviate the effects of the disease in other people. My wife is a peer counselor for the MS Society and I facilitate spouse groups. The primary motive is to make something good happen out of the tragedy of the disease by passing on our experience to those just starting out; somehow your problem becomes less when you can help someone else. Some of the most caring and generous people I have met have been the members of families in which there is a chronic, progressive disease.

Unfortunately you also get involved because you realize in a very fundamental way the crying lack of services for the chronically ill and you try to help fill the void in services that should be there except for lack of money and knowledge.

My wife's illness has expanded my horizons and I have learned a great deal. I have met many wonderful people and I have a renewed sense of direction and purpose in life. Transitional periods (and with chronic illness, one is always in transition) are also periods of new possibilities and growth. In one sense, we are all underachieving, only giving as much to life as our living demands of us; crises are a means of forcing us to develop capacities and strengths that might otherwise be dormant. I wish I could have accomplished this in some other way but we don't always have that choice.

There is a marvelous Zen saying that, "When the learner is ready, the teacher appears." These diseases, as awful as they are, are also in the deepest sense of the word, our teachers. I just hope I am up to the learning.

And when all is said and done, though Cari and I may have been dealt a "lousy hand," we still want to play it well.

CHAPTER 7

Cari's View

This chapter is called Cari's view: how I see the multiple sclerosis and how and in what way it has affected me, and also, as I've read through the chapters, it's become my reaction to how David sees me.

I have realized that his view of me is a very different one from what I had originally thought: I am seeing much more pain; I am seeing what, for me, seems to be much exaggeration of the condition that I view myself in. I am seeing myself much more as an invalid and, as I have often said, much more in-valid. I don't feel, although I am seeing through David's eyes that he *does* feel, that I am quite as helpless or quite as much of a burden, quite as much of an albatross around the neck. I somehow have never thought of myself as being so much on the mind and in the thoughts of those around me, so I have a double view here. I know how I feel about the way multiple sclerosis has affected me, and I am now getting a better appreciation of how I am affecting my most significant other, my husband, David.

I feel that my children's responses to the MS have all been very different. The youngest, Jim, casually handed me a paper he had written for his psychology course on Alfred Adler's theory of compensation, citing my way of dealing with the MS as an example. Jim's attitude is that he will help me any way he can, providing I take the initiative and do the asking.

My younger daughter, Emily, had also written a paper; hers was for an English course and explored causes of multiple sclerosis. She dropped it into a pile of papers I was going through, commenting rather brusquely that I might like to read it. Her way of handling the MS has been to quietly provide me with little aids: a lap board, light weights, warm slipper-socks, a soothing CD, pockets to put over the arm-rests of the wheelchair to carry small items like my keys and wallet, etc. Her husband, David, with the help of his father, has built a small ramp to enable me to get into their house.

Dan, my older son, professes to be totally uncon-cerned about the MS. It is he, however, who generally calls to check on me when David is out of town or when he hasn't heard from me in a few days. On a weekend after a snow, he will often appear, sometimes unan-nounced, to make sure that the front walk, the drive-way, and my chairlift are shoveled out. Dan has carried me up and down stairs to get to the bathroom or just to see new furnishings. It has become a matter-of-fact family affair: his wife, Patti, gives me super haircuts in the comfort of my wheelchair in my own home, and his son, Joshua, has been helping me fill my pill holder since before his third birthday.

Although both daughters have expressed aware-ness of the genetic factors in multiple sclerosis, it is my oldest, Alison, who verbalizes her feelings so poig-nantly. My first defense, of course, is to zero in on the exaggerations, the outright "never-happeneds". I must accept, however, that these are her perceptions of me; even without them, my feelings are of sadness and guilt. I was able-bodied enough when they were little;

now that they are young adults, I feel much less a part of their lives, very much as a factor of the MS and my inabilities. I wish that I could have done more with them, for instance, in the planning of their weddings or their early days of parenting.

And along with the guilt of being the reason for their upset, is the small nagging fear, which I work at pushing away, that any one of them might possibly inherit the combination of genes that would result in MS.

Language has always been very important to me. Words have to look and mean exactly what I want them to; sentences have to have a certain rhythm to them. Words like "disabled" grate against me. I am not disabled—a car is disabled; when you take all the wires out of a toaster, it might be disabled. I am a person: I am not disabled; I *have* a disability.

I am not handicapped, either. I am handicapped by the impediments put in my way either by nature, like mountains, which I can accept, or by people, like lack of curb cuts or poor facilities in the bathroom, which I find infinitely harder to accept; those handicapping impediments can and should be eliminated.

In like manner, co-disabled has for me the same connotation as co-dependent. Someone who is a co-dependent is aiding and abetting the alcoholic or drug user to use the drug or alcohol. Someone who is called co-disabled is hardly aiding and abetting anyone to have a disability: a co-disabler is certainly feeling the effects of the disability but hardly adding to it. I find that word, that attitude, difficult to accept.

Power and control are two important needs all through our lives. I see the desire for control in the negative behavior of the two-year-old who runs the other way when called and whose favorite word is "no", and again in the rebellious teenager who breaks curfews. I also see it in the frustrated rioting of oppressed people, and I definitely acknowledge it in my own behavior: the more the body part of me loses control, the more the mind part of me wants control even over the smallest things. A lived-in look to the home becomes an impediment to the wheels of my chair. The book that is thrown back into the recesses of the sofa with a coffee table blocking it might as well be on the moon if my reacher is not long enough to retrieve it. A chair that has been moved for conversation becomes an obstacle for my getting through a room. Food put back in the refrigerator and dishes put back on shelves need to be returned to specific places so that I can retrieve them easily by myself and retain as much independence as possible. I need control over these small things.

Maintaining my independence is very important to me, and most of my frustration comes from the times when I cannot be as independent as I want. It takes me much longer to finish even the smallest task than it ever did before. There are some tasks, of course, that I can not do at all. I weigh my dependency needs very carefully, doing whatever I can myself even though it might take longer. It takes me longer for activities ranging from taking my shower and getting dressed in the morning to preparing dinner and cleaning up in the evening. I want to maintain as much independence as possible for as long as possible.

As my physical abilities erode, so too does the range of my activities. I can no longer walk, therefore I cannot get into certain places. I can no longer transfer easily from my scooter into my car, getting my legs up and under the wheel, so I cannot drive. This means my excursions are more at the whim of others. My friends have been wonderful about transporting me in my car to restaurants and the theater with them; they have even carried me in my chair up stairs into some houses. When I have to go any place else locally I call on THE RIDE which is special transportation for people with disabilities. This means, however, a three-day reservation in advance. Spontaneity is no longer the name of the game.

"Don't call David" and "C'mon, you can do it" have become my mantras as I exhort myself and the particular non-compliant body parts to cooperate and do what I need done—move, not buckle under me, hold a pen, etc. (I also curse a little.)

The frustrations are very great, and yet I can take pride in the accomplishments, too: when I can dress myself in a shorter time than I have done before, when I can get my socks and shoes off or on more easily or faster, when I can empty the dishwasher and put most of the dishes back on the shelves in the cupboards, when I can transfer with no difficulty from one chair to another, or when I work and work at a transfer and finally complete it—for all these little things I first thank the Powers-that-be and then feel a personal pride in that accomplishment. I also feel a sadness that I feel the pride for an action that for anyone else would be so insignificant. For me, though, it's my marathon.

Besides feelings of powerlessness, frustration, and disbelief that this is really happening to me, another feeling stemming from my having multiple sclerosis is one of gratitude. I am, of course grateful that the MS symptoms didn't become too debilitating until I had finished bringing up my children. I was able to be mobile as a mother of young children and do things with them and for them, and for that I am really grateful.

I am also grateful for the friends who have kept me in their circle and have made my home the focus of meetings and get-togethers. I am thankful for those friends who have been coming now for about two years, taking turns going through an exercise program with me so that my body will remain as strong and flexible as it possibly can. I am sure that it is because of them that the progression of the MS has been as slow as it has been. These friends come and exercise my leg and, more than that, they give of themselves: first and foremost, they are friends and it is wonderful to see a different one every day. We exercise, we talk, and we share, and I am grateful for that.

I get angry sometimes that I must be grateful. It would be nice to be grateful on ones own, but perhaps this is reminding me that there are many wonderful things and people in life. We have a beautiful new bedroom from which I can watch the birds and see my husband's garden. We really wouldn't have built the room if I could have continued to go upstairs; so I'm grateful for the room, and in a way, I have to be grateful that the MS pushed us into building it. I am grateful that I have had to take it a bit slower in life because there is not much choice when your body won't move quickly. Perhaps it is important for all of us to take time to smell the roses. I sit at our bedroom window and watch the birds at our feeder and the ever-changing vista of David's garden, and for this I am most grateful.

And, needless to say, perhaps, therefore, extremely important to say, I am most grateful to be with David in our marriage. Perhaps it can be considered a perfect marriage because it has not been perfected. The MS adds an extra challenge that we have to work at constantly—together.

I would not wish multiple sclerosis on anyone. That is not what I mean at all, and yet having MS has not been the end of the world. It has been the end of a world as I knew it, yet it has opened up another, different one with its own positives and negatives. This world is less stable, less certain, less predictable; this world forces me to keep focused on the here-and-now: no regrets for yesterday, no fears for tomorrow, only living in today.

Addendum

This book has been written over several years and because chronic, progressive illness does not stay still, some of the references to my own life situation are now obsolete. As of this writing (late 1994), Cari returned from a three week stay in a Rehabilitation Hospital in 1992. One leg has persistent contractures and consequently, she cannot stand; transferring from wheelchair to bed to toilet is very difficult. The doctors have told her that she will not walk again and they and she are devising ways to ensure that she will continue to make the transfers. She has not driven in over two years now and it is problematic whether she will ever be able to drive again. This loss is immense.

Through it all, Cari keeps plugging away—every so often, as I do, wondering what we are doing here and how we got to this place. Sadness may not be the right word for it; at times it feels like despair for both of us. And yet, there is so much good here too. The outpouring of letters and visits from friends and relatives has been immense. Our children have been very helpful and supportive. We still manage to take our trips downtown, Cari riding and me walking, to eat out in a restaurant. We still enjoy watching movies on the VCR and the visits from our friends and family. Our grandson, Joshua, age 3, is a source of joy as he helps to push his grandmother in her manual chair and rides with her in the electric wheelchair; there is no loss for him.

Cari recently participated in a television program highlighting the Americans with Disability Act and she demonstrated how inaccessible so much of our society is to the physically disabled. Neither of us knows what the future holds for us as we ratchet down the disability path, but we do know we will do this one together.

References

1. Strong, M. *Mainstay*. Boston, MA. Little, Brown Co., 1988.
2. Cluff, L. Chronic Disease and the Quality of Care. *J of Chronic Diseases* 34:299–304, 1981.
3. Nuland, S.D. *How We Die*. New York, Knopf. 1994.
4. Sager, C. *Marriage Contracts and Couple Theory*. New York, Rawson Wade, Inc., 1978.
5. Ewtmacher, P., Bostic, E., and Harris, M. *Economic Impact of Diabetes*. N.I.H. Publication #85–1468.
6. Wasow, M. Chronic Schizophrenia and Alzheimer's Disease: The Loss for Parents, Spouses, and Children Compared. *J of Chronic Diseases* 38, #8, 711–16. 1985
7. Zahn, M. Incapacity, Impotence and Invisible Impairment. *J of Health and Social Behavior* 14: 115–123. 1993.
8. Minuchin, S. *Families and Family Therapy*. Cambridge, MA 1978.
9. Roy, R. *Consequences of Parental Illness on Children: A Review. Social Work and Social Sciences Review* 2(2) 109–121. 1990.
10. Rabins, P. Management of Dementia in the Family Context. *Psychosomatics*, 25:369–375. 1984.
11. Matson and Brooks. Adjusting to Multiple Sclerosis: An Explorative Study. *Social Science and Medicine* 11:245–50. 1977.
12. Pearlin and Schooler. The Structure of Coping. *J of Health and Social Behavior* 19:2–21. 1978.
13. Dundon, M., Cramer, S., Novak, C. Distress and Cop-

ing Among Caregivers of Victims of Alzheimer's Disease. Paper Presented at the American Psychological Asociation. New York City. August, 1987.

14. Silverstein, S. *The Giving Tree*. New York, Harper and Row, 1964.
15. Kushner. *When Bad Things Happen to Good People*. New York: Avon Books, 1983.

Appendix

A. Multiple Sclerosis

Multiple sclerosis is a central nervous system disease in which the myelin sheath protecting nerves in the brain and spinal cord become scarred (sclerotic) and thereby distort the transmission of nerve impulses. The disease was first described by the French neurologist Jean-Martin Charlot in the latter half of the nineteenth century.

Multiple sclerosis is an auto-immune disease in which the white blood cells (T-cells) attack the myelin sheath surrounding the nerve fiber. Myelin serves on the nerve fiber much like insulation on an electrical cord. Without it, the nerve is unable to transmit impulses efficiently, and as a result, transmission may be either delayed or cease completely. Since demyelinization can occur in any of the brain's areas of white matter, a variety of functions may be affected, thereby making the diagnosis difficult. Symptoms frequently include one or more of the following: muscle weakness, numbness, spasticity, fatigue, vision problems, paralysis, and bladder, bowel, and sexual dysfunction.

About 250,000 Americans are thought to have MS, with approximately 9,000 new cases diagnosed each year. It is the most common cause of neurological disability that attacks persons between the ages of 15 and 55 with peak frequency of onset occurring at about age 30. It is more prevalent in cold climates than warm, more common in women than men, and more common in whites than blacks or Asians. The illness has a tendency to run in families; siblings of a person with MS have a 10 to 15 times higher risk than the general population of getting MS while 50 percent of identical twin pairs were concordant for the disease—that is, both twins ended up with the disease. Daughters of mothers with MS have the highest risk of developing the disease: 5 percent. The risk for the general population is 0.1 percent. MS is not considered as being directly inherited; more likely than not, the disease is the result of an inherited susceptibility that is affected by environmental factors. It is not known what environmental forces will ignite the genetic fuse; the suspicion is that a virus somehow alters the composition of the T-cells so that they now attack the myelin sheath. The origin of the disease may be infectious but MS is not contagious.

There is no medically recognized cure for the disease although there are many claims of cures. Because of the remitting nature of the disease, many therapies seem effective on a given patient because of a remission of symptoms which might have spontaneously occurred anyway.

A number of drugs have been used both singly and in combination in the treatment of the symptoms of MS. Steroid drugs, which reduce inflammation, are a mainstay of current MS therapy. Experimental drugs which aim to suppress the body's immune system have been tried. Among these is the anticancer drug, Cytoxan. Another drug, Imuran, has shown some benefit in patients who suffer frequent flare-ups of the disease; a drug currently being tested is Copolymer I which seems to reduce the frequency of exacerbation but does not affect the ultimate clinical outcome of the disease. Not only does the remitting nature of the disease prevent clear data from emerging from the clinical studies, but so many of the symptoms of MS are subjective in nature that improvement cannot be documented even though the patient feels better—the placebo effect is very great with this disease.

The course of the disease varies markedly: about 20 percent of patients have a benign form of the disease in which they experience one or two mild attacks (called exacerbations) that do not recur and leave no disability. Another 20 to 30 percent have exacerbating-remitting disease with long intervals between attacks and symptoms that disappear partially or totally in the interim. The largest group, about 40 percent, have remitting progressive disease in which the symptoms do not disappear completely and get progressively worse after each attack. Another 10 to 20 percent of patients have chronic progressive disease: the rate of decline is steady although it (the rate) may vary from individual to individual. Multiple sclerosis is rarely terminal.

B. Alzheimer's Disease

In 1907, Alois Alzheimer, a physician in the Insane Asylum in Frankfurt, observed a 51-year-old woman who had impaired memory, could not find her way around her own apartment, was paranoid, and could not remember the names of simple objects. She was institutionalized, gradually deteriorated, and died four-and-a-half years later. On autopsy, Alzheimer found her brain to be grossly atrophied with a great deal of cortical cell loss, and a very large number of senile plaques on the neural fibers. (Senile plaques are minute areas of tissue degeneration and demyelinization. They are present in normal aging brains, but in Alzheimer's disease [hereafter referred to as AD], the number of neuritic plaques grossly exceed the norm for that age group.) Also noted by Alzheimer, were the presence of neurofibriliary tangles. These tangles, which occur only in humans, are composed of badly disorganized tubular and fibriliary elements of the neuron. In a normal neuron, the neurotubules make up the skeleton of the cell running from the body to the axons and dendrites. They seem to provide both structural integrity of the cell and to serve as a transportation network for the movement of hormones that are responsible for transmission of the neural impulses. A definite diagnosis of Alzheimer's disease as seen on an autopsy would involve both an abnormally large number of neuritic plaques and the presence of the neurofibriliary tangles.

It is difficult to determine just how prevalent AD is because relatively few cases come to autopsy where the definitive diagnosis can be made; estimates in hospital populations vary from 20 to 60 percent of all adult patients with progressive dementia. It is also reckoned that there are anywhere from 1.5 million to 4 million Americans who have the disease. (One study has estimated that 22 percent of people over the age of 80 may have the disease.) All investigators agree that it is the most common cause of senile dementia and that its incidence is on the rise as our population ages. For many years researchers designated any dementia that occurred before age 65 as Alzheimer's and after age 65 as senile dementia. Current thinking is that this may be the same disease.

The cause of AD is unknown. There is evidence of a genetic factor. A Swedish study found that primary relatives of Alzheimer's patients have approximately a four-fold greater risk of developing the disease than the general population. This is true only for early onset Alzheimer's (before age 65) and is not so for late onset of the disease. A recently conducted study of twins has found that if one twin had AD, there was a 40 to 50 percent chance that the other one would develop it as well. This was true for both fraternal and identical twins. The fact that identical twins who are genetically manacled have less than a 50 percent chance of both developing AD supports the notion of contributing environmental factors. Moreover, investigators found that the age of the disease onset could vary as much as 13 years from twin to twin. This would strongly indicate both a genetic and an environmental basis for the disease.

One striking feature of AD is its relationship to Downs syndrome. Almost all people with Downs syndrome develop AD if they reach age thirty-five or above. Conversely, there is a six-fold greater likelihood of finding a Downs syndrome family member among the relatives of Alzheimer's patients than in a control population which has no AD patients.

It is beginning to look as though some individuals may be born with a genetic defect leading to AD that does not get expressed unless there is some environmental trigger. Among possible environmental culprits suggested have been stress, toxins, and immunological factors such as a slow virus. Investigators have tried to determine if an infectious agent, such as an exotic virus, is the cause, but to date there is no evidence that AD is transmissible. Aluminum toxicity and head injuries have also been investigated.

The results of all studies on the cause have been equivocal; and few, if any, investigators think that brain injuries or aluminum toxicity could be more than a contributing factor. The disease process is almost certainly complex and probably involves several different factors.

The disease usually begins after age 50. Death is generally 5 to 12 years after onset although individual patients have been known to live 20 years; others deteriorate rapidly and die within one or two years of the diagnosis.

Although the causes of AD are shrouded in mystery, the clinical course of the disease is quite clear. Patients with this disease undergo progressive intellectual deterioration. Remissions do not occur and plateau periods of arrested progression are seldom seen. The course is steadily downhill and only the rate of progression varies from patient to patient. It's as though the hands of the developmental clock turn counterclockwise ultimately leaving the patient where he started in life as a dependent infant.

The onset of the disease is usually quite subtle and always involves memory loss. Since the personality and social behavior remain intact for several years, the patient is frequently able to hide his or her deficiencies from most people which often leads them to underestimate the difficulty or to excuse it. As the disease progresses, judgment is affected with patients being unable to reason through problems. Spatial and temporal disorientations also occur in the early stages, and patients are often found wandering lost in places that used to be quite familiar to them. With further progression, there is increased memory loss, restlessness, and further spatial disorientation; hallucinations are quite common. In the final stages, intellectual functions are severely deteriorated and patients generally die of pneumonia or of urinary tract infections.

C. Diabetes

Ask someone to locate the islets of Langerhans and you will receive a wide range of answers, seldom the right one. The most likely response is off the coast of Denmark; in actuality, they are found within the pancreas, a gland that weighs about eight ounces and is situated below and behind the stomach. It is the failure of the beta cells of the islets to produce insulin which causes diabetes. The beta cells, when stimulated by glucose as well as other foods in the diet, release insulin. Insulin is the main messenger and mobilizer of the fuels (glucose, protein, and fat) contained within the food we eat. Each normal pancreas has about 100,000 islets of Langerhans and each islet contains 80 to 100 beta cells. In a marvelously precise mechanism, which is still not completely understood, these cells are capable of monitoring the blood glucose level; within 60 to 90 seconds they can deliver any amount of insulin necessary for the body to function. In nondiabetics, the pancreas releases just enough insulin to enable the body to use food as energy and to store the excess nutrients in the liver and muscles. Insulin operates as a traffic policeman directing the nutrients from food into the appropriate uses and maintaining the blood glucose level within a rather narrow normal range (50 to 100mg percent of blood after fasting and never above 150mg percent after a meal or after a glucose challenge).

In diabetics, a nonfunctioning pancreas results in an insulin shortage. Consequently, the blood levels of glucose and fat are elevated. Normally the kidneys would retrieve the excess glucose; in diabetes there is so much extra glucose that it spills into the urine much like water going over a dam. (The Indian name for diabetes is "Madhumeha" or "honey urine"; the Latin word "Mellitus," [honey] was used later.) When fuel provided by the food nutrients cannot be utilized by the body cells because of the low level of insulin available, the sensation of hunger appears and the individual overeats, (polyphagia). Since the food is still not available to the body, the individual will be tired and weak; because there is so much spill-over of glucose into the urine, there will be excessive water loss through the frequent urinations and the person will become chronically thirsty (polydipsia). The classic symptoms then for untreated diabetes are tiredness, weakness, loss of weight, frequent urination, excessive thirst, and hunger. The diagnosis of diabetes mellitus, however, must be confirmed by blood and urine glucose tests.

There are two major forms of diabetes: juvenile-onset and maturity-onset. In juvenile-onset diabetes, the symptoms usually occur rapidly and dramatically because the beta cells produce almost no insulin. Juvenile-onset diabetes is not confined to young persons (under age 40); 15 percent to 20 percent of all older diabetics have the juvenile form of the disease. In maturity-onset diabetes, on the other hand, the symptoms occur gradually. The beta cells usually produce some insulin and consequently there are milder symptoms. The typical maturity-onset diabetic is obese and develops the disease after the age of 40, although 5 percent of diabetics under the age of twenty have the maturity-onset type of diabetes. Maturity-onset diabetes can very often be treated by dietary restriction. In normal persons the body is able to produce just enough insulin to match the fuel supplied by eating. By restricting the food intake, there is a better use of the available insulin and there is less demand for the manufacture of more insulin. Juvenile-onset diabetics, however, must receive injections of insulin to replace the vastly depleted or nonexistent levels of insulin in their bodies.

Prior to 1921, most juvenile-onset diabetics died, literally wasting away, their bodies unable to utilize the energy provided by the food they ate. In 1921 Banting and Best in Ontario, Canada began a landmark series of studies in the treatment of diabetes. When minced and purified islet tissue from dead animals was injected into live animals with diabetes, the blood sugar levels fell, thus demonstrating that diabetes can be controlled. The injection of insulin does not replace the very sensitive monitoring function provided by the body's natural glucose regulating mechanism. Injected insulin jolts the body and it is difficult to maintain the glucose level within the narrow, normal range; intermittent, injected insulin provides no cure for diabetes nor does it alter the diabetic state.

There is a genetic component present in diabetes that seems to be expressed by some environmental "stressors." There is no single gene theory that can explain the inheritance of diabetes; for example, even if both parents are diabetic, the children have only a 30 percent chance of becoming diabetic. Twelve percent of newly diagnosed diabetics have close relatives with diabetes, whereas only two percent of normal individuals in the general population have relatives with diabetes. Maturity-onset diabetes has a similar genetic component with the added factor that obesity is probably the single most influential environmental factor.

Other causes of diabetes that have been suggested are hormonal imbalances, drugs and medication, and illness that affects the pancreas and ultimately the beta cells. In short, diabetes appears to be a disease that is multicausal, and there are probably several etiological factors yet to be discovered.

There are two very dangerous acute complications that can occur when maintenance is not well established: hypoglycemia and ketoacidosis. Hypoglycemia is a condition of low blood sugar level (less than 50mg percent) that occurs when the individual takes too much insulin, when there is an insufficient food intake, or when the person exercises too much. When this occurs, the diabetic experiences hunger, nausea, weakness, and confusion. If treatment is delayed, unconsciousness may occur. The treatment for hypoglycemia is sugar or glucose in some form.

The flip side of hypoglycemia is ketoacidosis which is too high a blood sugar level caused by too much food, too little exercise, and too little insulin. As the blood sugar level rises, the body loses fluid and the person dehydrates. Because there is no fuel available from the food, the body begins to break down fats. Ketone bodies are the end products of improper fat breakdown and these spill over into the urine. As the patient becomes dehydrated, coma and unconsciousness occur. Treatment requires the injection of insulin and the rehydration of the body. The diabetic must always steer a tricky course between the Scylla of hypoglycemia (low blood sugar) and the Charybdis of ketoacidosis (high blood sugar), both of which can result in death if not treated properly.

The terror of diabetes lies not so much with the disease itself, which in many cases can be controlled by rigid adherence to a diet and exercise program and to the timely injections of insulin, but in the possibility of complications from the diabetes that can occur despite good maintenance.

The mechanism for the development of complications is not well understood but the statistics are rather grim. Long-term diabetics tend to develop problems of vision (retinopathy) and diabetes is one of the main causes of partial visual loss in the United States. Twenty-five percent of all juvenile-onset diabetics between the age of 30 and 50 will become legally blind; 30 to 40 percent of insulin dependent diabetics will develop disease serious enough to end in kidney failure. Diabetics are twice as prone to coronary heart disease as are non-diabetics—75 percent of the deaths of diabetics are due to heart failure as opposed to 50 percent in the general population. Diabetes causes about 50 percent of all amputations of the foot and leg among adults. Maternal diabetes is a leading cause of fetal death; it is estimated that there are 341,000 deaths every year directly attributed to diabetes and 100,000 to its complications. A frequent complication of diabetes is neuropathy sometimes referred to as "diabetic neuritis." The symptoms can affect any nerve pathway in the body producing a wide variety of debilitating symptoms. Diabetics have twice as many disabilities as non-diabetics. Diabetics have on the average three times the health care expense as the general population. The total direct medical care expense for diabetics in 1977 was 6.9 billion. The total overall expense of diabetes in the United States was estimated at 14 billion dollars. This figure has gone to over 20 billion for 1987 and is rising.

Diabetes appears to be on the rise as our population ages and people live long enough to develop the disease. In the past 6 years, 3.6 million new cases have been diagnosed, about 10 percent of them children. One in every 20 persons in the United States is now affected by diabetes. It is a formidable disease.

D. Arthritis

Like multiple sclerosis, arthritis is an auto-immune disease. In the case of rheumatoid arthritis, the white blood cells attack the linings of the joints, causing severe inflammation. Arthritis is actually many diseases, all of which involve an inflammation of connective tissue in the body. These diseases include gout, lupus, scleroderma, and osteoarthritis (the most common form of arthritis and one generally seen in the elderly populations). Rheumatoid arthritis, which affects over two million Americans, is the most common form of arthritis of younger people and is the disease we will consider here.

Rheumatoid arthritis is first of all a systemic disease that affects all parts of the body, generally starting as feelings of fatigue, loss of appetite, weakness, and a generalized aching and stiffness. As the disease progresses, the pain begins to be localized in particular joints in which there is stiffness and increasing limitation of movement. In a normal joint the terminal points of the bone are covered with smooth, protective cartilage and the entire joint is enclosed in a capsule lined with a layer of cells called the synovium. The cartilage is the weight-bearing surface of the joint, and the synovial cells secrete a fluid that lubricates the joints and enables the cartilage to move freely.

In a normally functioning joint the friction is so low that the cartilage is never subject to stress. In a rheumatoid joint the synovium becomes thickened and inflamed; during flare-up of the disease the joint swells as the amount of fluid increases. The connective tissue of the joint becomes the field on which the battles of arthritis are fought. Thus, the joint becomes very painful and movement very difficult. Long-term rheumatoid joints show a build-up of the synovial tissue which erodes the cartilage, reducing the firm smooth surface of the cartilage to a rough, pitted one; eventually the bone is exposed. When this happens, the joint becomes a bone on bone junction and is extremely painful to move as bone grinds against bone.

What causes the white blood cells to attack the synovium of the joint is unknown. The disease is much more prevalent in women than men. In people under the age of 60, there are 5 times as many women affected as men. After age 60, the ratio is almost equal. Arthritis usually goes in remission during pregnancy but generally show exacerbation postpartum. There is a tendency for arthritis to run in families but the genetic component is not strong.

Treatment of the disease is generally confined to reducing the inflammation through anti-inflammatory drugs such as aspirin and cortisone derivatives, and controlling pain. Where the joint has been destroyed by disease, surgical replacement may be indicated. At first the flare-ups are intermittent, but become more sustained with time. The clinical course is generally downward, with increasing pain and loss of mobility.

In addition to the potential loss of mobility, the hallmark of arthritis is pain. There is pain felt in joints during the flare-ups of the disease and there is the chronic, never-ending pain when a joint is destroyed by the disease. A friend of mine who has rheumatoid arthritis has written about her pain:

At times I have felt like there have been tidal waves of pain and tiredness breaking over me and I just start to catch my breath after one, and another one comes breaking down any sort of wall I have quickly tried to build. At other times I have felt like a rudderless ship on the ocean in a storm. After the peak of the flare-up, I couldn't face anybody. I felt war-wounded and had to have time to recover.

E. Lupus

Systemic lupus erythematosus (SLE) or, lupus, as it is commonly known, is a chronic, inflammatory disease that may affect joints, kidneys, lungs, nervous system, skin, or any of a number of other organs of the body. Lupus, Latin for wolf, was named for the erosive facial rash that is characteristic of the disease: the damage to the skin caused by the rash was likened to the devastations caused by the attack of a hungry wolf. Erythematosus refers to the scaly, red rash that looks like an open butterfly on both cheeks and the bridge of the nose, and occurs after exposure to the sun; in actuality this particular butterfly rash occurs in a little less than half of all patients diagnosed with SLE.

Lupus is an auto-immune disease in which the individual develops antibodies to his or her own tissue, referred to medically as a loss of self-tolerance. This chronic, internal civil war can be fought in any of a number of areas of the body causing a bewildering array of symptoms that makes the diagnosis of lupus difficult. The disease can also have many different courses, ranging from very mild to very severe and in rare cases can be rapidly fatal. In most cases the disease follows a chronic, irregular course with long periods of complete or near complete remission, which increases immensely the difficulty of making a diagnosis. Current medical thinking is that SLE is not a single disease but rather a group of closely related diseases with a distinct genetic, immunologic, and pathological bases. Because SLE can and does effect many different places in the body, it is very difficult to diagnose.

The most common clinical manifestations of SLE follow:

Joint involvement is present in over 90 percent of all lupus patients and frequently lupus patients are initially diagnosed as having arthritis. There is swelling of the joints and pain in movement, most commonly of the fingers, hands, wrists, knees, and ankles. It is nonerosive arthritis—more of an arthralgia. Rarely is there permanent damage to a joint.

Abnormalities of the skin, hair, and mucous membranes are the second most common manifestation of SLE, occurring in about 85 percent of all diagnosed patients. Patients show raised red rashes on the skin: some with the classic butterfly rash (42%) and others with discoid rashes that become permanently scarring in older lesions giving a devastated appearance to the skin. The rashes become evident after exposure to the sun. There is frequently patchy hair loss (27%), as well as oral ulcers (12%). Kidney involvement is present in over half of the patients (53%), and inflammation of the linings of the lungs (pleurisy, 45%) and heart (pericarditis, 27%) are also fairly common. Lupus can affect the neurological system by causing inflammation in any one part of it and producing varied symptoms including seizures and psychosis.

A positive blood test indicating the presence of ANA, antibodies of the cell nuclei, is almost always present in the active phase of lupus. ANA are also present in other auto-immune diseases, so that a positive ANA test does not in itself indicate the presence of lupus. Other common complaints of lupus patients are fatigue, weight loss, and fever in the absence of any obvious infections.

SLE is a disease that affects approximately 500,000 Americans, mainly occurring in young women between the ages of twenty and forty. Women are nine times more likely to have lupus than men, and black women are three times more likely to have it than white women. The cause of the disease is unknown, although there appears to be a genetic component that is triggered by environmental stresses. The triggers in lupus are thought to be viral infections, ultraviolet light, drugs, pregnancy, and stress. Immune system abnormalities appear in up to 10 percent of relatives of patients with SLE, and they are present in less than 1 percent of the general population. Children of lupus parents have a 1-in-20 chance of getting lupus, while the prevalence rate for young women is 1 in 700. The overall incidence rate for lupus is approximately 1 in 2,000 in the general population. Viral infections in genetically predisposed individuals have been implicated in all auto-immune diseases. The virus appears to alter the genetic structure of the white blood cells so that they become "intolerant to the self" (in MS the white blood cells attack the myelin sheath of the nerves; in lupus and rheumatoid arthritis, it is mainly the connective tissues of the body). Ultraviolet light, by causing damage to the DNA structure in the cells, invokes an auto-immune response in the patient that often causes the characteristic lupus butterfly rash. Over half of all lupus patients have some photo sensitivity.

Drugs such as hydralazine, procainamide, and possibly hydantoin, often cause lupus-like symptoms that disappear when the use of the drugs is discontinued. Penicillin and sulfonamides are drugs that were sometimes used to control infections associated with lupus; they also seem to exacerbate SLE. Patients and doctors have to be very careful as to what drugs and combinations of drugs are used in treating the disease symptoms.

Until recently, the natural course of untreated SLE was considered to be very bleak. The prognosis seems to be improving greatly. In 1956 patients were given only a 50 percent chance of surviving four years. Today, they have a better than 90 percent chance of surviving at least ten years. Prognosis for patients having kidney involvement and/or nervous system damage is poorer.

There is no cure for lupus. Treatment is directed at the disease activity and is designed to prevent inflammation and permanent organ damage. Anti-inflammatory drugs, such as steroids and salicylates are generally used to control the inflammation process, and the anti-malarial drug, chloroquine, is frequently used to control the discoid skin rash. Antibiotics but not penicillin or sulfonamides, are used to control any systemic infection. Almost all of these drugs have unpleasant side effects and must be administered under careful medical supervision. Because of the exacerbating/remitting nature of the disease, it is never known whether the treatment was effective or the symptoms would have disappeared anyway. All in all, lupus is a puzzling and frightening disease.

Additional copies of *In the Shadows* may be ordered for $19.95 plus $2.00 shipping and handling.

Please print

Name _____

Street_____ Apt.#____

City _____ State _____ Zip _____

Mail to:
     Jade Press
     Box 822
     Bedford, MA 01730

Include $21.95 for each copy of
In the Shadows.

Please cut along dotted line